Nutritional information disclaimer: We have provided nutritional information for these recipes. The calculations were done using online tools. Even though we have tried to provide accurate nutritional information, these figures should be considered estimates. Various factors (such as product types or brands, natural fluctuations in fresh produce, substitutions, serving sizes, and the way ingredients are processed) can change the nutritional factors in any given

recipe. To obtain the most accurate representation of the nutritional information in a given recipe, please calculate the nutritional information with the actual ingredients and amounts used, using your preferred nutrition calculator. Under no circumstances shall Ketoveo be responsible for any loss or damage resulting from your reliance on the given nutritional information. You are solely responsible for ensuring that any nutritional information provided is accurate, complete, and useful.

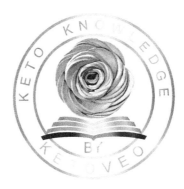

Go to **www.ketoveo.com** for more guides and resources to help you on your keto journey.

CONTENTS

FLU SMOOTHIE

Servings: 1

Nutritional Facts Per Serving:

| Net Carbs: | 7.7 g | Protein: | 3.3 g |
| Fat: | 9.4 g | Calories: | 148 kcal |

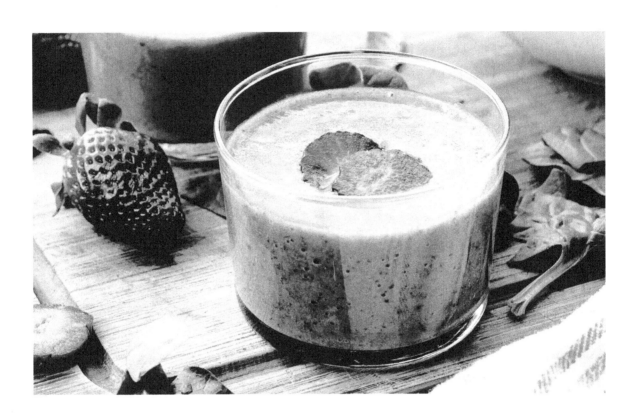

INGREDIENTS

½ cup kale

2 large strawberries

Half avocado

½ cup cucumber with peel

½ cup unsweetened almond milk

1 tsp Swerve or sweetener of choice

1 tsp sugar-free vanilla extract

½ tsp sea salt

This is how you make the recipe

1. Add all ingredients to a blender. Blend until smooth.

2. Chill or pour over ice.

3. Serve and enjoy!

CUCUMBER GREEN TEA DETOX SMOOTHIE

Servings: 2

Nutritional Facts Per Serving:
Net Carbs:	2.35 g	Protein:	0.9 g
Fat:	4.45 g	Calories:	56 kcal

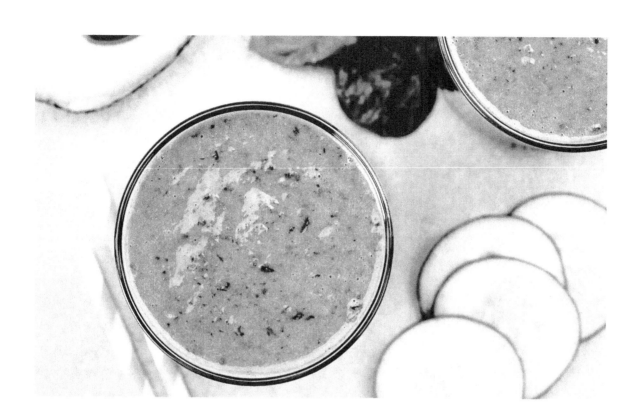

INGREDIENTS

1 cup water
2 tsp matcha green tea powder
1 cup sliced cucumber
⅓ cup avocado slices
1 tsp lemon juice
½ tsp Swerve or sweetener of choice
½ cup ice cubes

This is how you make the recipe

1. Pour the water and green tea powder into a blender first and give it a whirl to combine.

2. Add the remaining ingredients and blend on high until smooth.

3. Taste and adjust sweetener as desired.

4. Serve and enjoy!

PEANUT BUTTER CHOCOLATE MILKSHAKE

Servings: 1

Nutritional Facts Per Serving:
Net Carbs: 4.83 g   Protein: 5.6 g
Fat: 5.6 g   Calories: 165 kcal

INGREDIENTS

1 cup unsweetened coconut milk
1 tbsp unsweetened cocoa powder
1 tbsp unsweetened peanut butter
Sweetener of your choice to taste
Pinch of sea salt

This is how you make the recipe

1. Place all ingredients in blender.

2. Blend until well combined and frothy.

3. Serve and enjoy!

CREAMY CINNAMON SMOOTHIE

Servings: 1

Nutritional Facts Per Serving:

| Net Carbs: | 8.9 g | Protein: | 50 g |
| Fat: | 41 g | Calories: | 622 kcal |

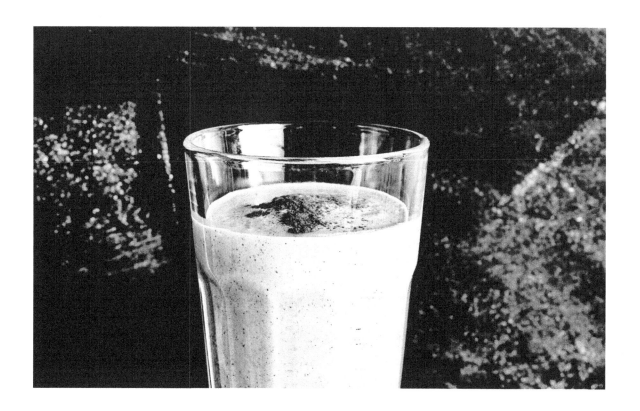

INGREDIENTS

½ cup coconut milk

½ cup water & few ice cubes

1 tbsp MCT oil or coconut oil

½ tsp cinnamon

1 tbsp ground chia seeds

¼ cup plain or vanilla unsweetened protein powder or egg white protein powder

This is how you make the recipe

1. Add the coconut milk, protein powder, cinnamon and ground chia seeds in a blender.

2. Add the MCT oil or coconut oil, water and ice. If you use coconut oil, make sure you blend it well.

3. Add ice and, if you want some sweetness , add sweetener of your choice.

4. Blend until smooth and enjoy!

FRUIT-FREE SMOOTHIE

Servings: 1

Nutritional Facts Per Serving:

Net Carbs:	8.1 g	Protein:	26 g
Fat:	29 g	Calories:	430 kcal

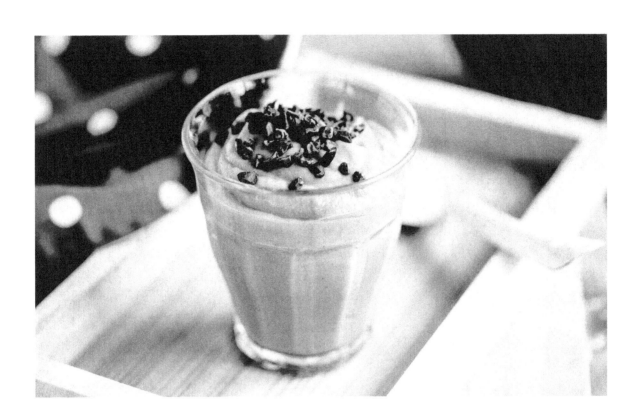

INGREDIENTS

1 cup unsweetened almond milk

½ avocado

1-2 cups spinach

½ scoop keto protein powder

1 tsp cocoa powder

1 tbsp MCT oil

½ tsp Swerve or sweetener of choice

¼ - ½ cup water for thinning out to desired consistency

Ice cubes

1 tsp cacao nibs (optional)

This is how you make the recipe

1. Add all the ingredients except cacao nibs into a blender and blend on high until smooth.

2. Pour into a glass and sprinkle with cacao nibs.

3. Serve and enjoy!

MILKSHAKE SMOOTHIE WITH RASPBERRIES

Servings: 2

Nutritional Facts Per Serving:

Net Carbs:	5.8 g	Protein:	2 g
Fat:	14.5 g	Calories:	164.5 kcal

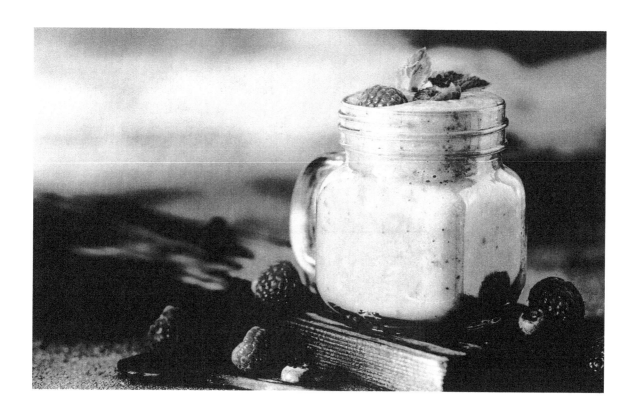

INGREDIENTS

1 cup unsweetened plain almond milk

1 cup crushed ice

¼ cup heavy whipping cream

¼ cup fresh raspberries

2 tbsp Swerve or sweetener of choice

1 tbsp cream cheese

½ tsp sugar-free vanilla extract

Pinch of sea salt

This is how you make the recipe

1. Microwave cream cheese in a small bowl for about 5 seconds or until soft.

2. Add all ingredients to a blender. Blend until very smooth.

3. Taste and adjust accordingly by adding more Swerve for a sweeter taste, or another tablespoon of cream cheese for a creamier finish.

4. Serve and enjoy!

BLUEBERRY COCONUT CHIA SMOOTHIES

Servings: 4

Nutritional Facts Per Serving:

Net Carbs:	26.5 g	Protein:	7 g
Fat:	18.75 g	Calories:	309.3 kcal

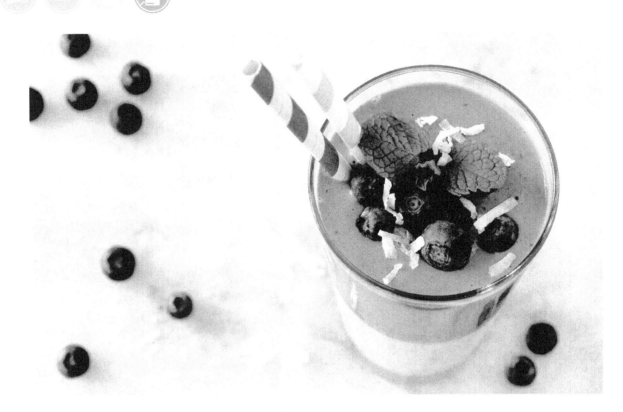

INGREDIENTS

1 cup fresh blueberries

1 cup full-fat Greek yogurt (use almond milk or coconut milk yogurt for dairy-free and vegan option)

½ cup coconut cream (the really thick creamy stuff from the top of the can of full-fat coconut milk)

1 cup unsweetened almond milk

2 tbsp coconut oil

2 tbsp ground chia seed

2 tbsp Swerve or sweetener of choice

You can add protein powder, collagen or any other supplement that appeals to you (optional)

This is how you make the recipe

1. Combine all ingredients in blender and blend until smooth.

2. Divide among 4 glasses and enjoy!

SALTED CARAMEL SMOOTHIE

Servings: 1

Nutritional Facts Per Serving:

Net Carbs:	3.1 g	Protein:	1.9 g
Fat:	27 g	Calories:	261 kcal

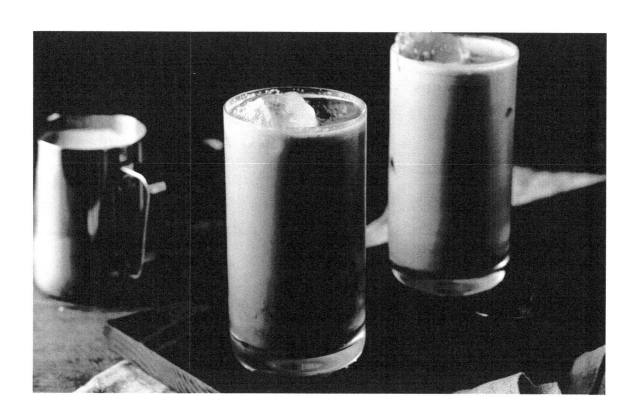

INGREDIENTS

1 bag Bigelow Salted Caramel Tea steeped in 6 oz. water

1 cup unsweetened almond milk

2 tbsp whipping cream

1 tbsp MCT oil

1 tsp Swerve or sweetener of choice

¾ tsp xanthan gum

8 ice cubes

This is how you make the recipe

1. Steep 1 bag of Bigelow Salted Caramel Tea in 6 oz. water. Remove and discard tea bag when done.

2. Combine remaining ingredients in a blender and blend until smooth.

3. Pour into a glass and enjoy!

HEALTHY CHOCOLATE PEANUT BUTTER SMOOTHIE

Servings: 3

Nutritional Facts Per Serving:

Net Carbs:	8.3 g	Protein:	8.7 g
Fat:	41 g	Calories:	431.7 kcal

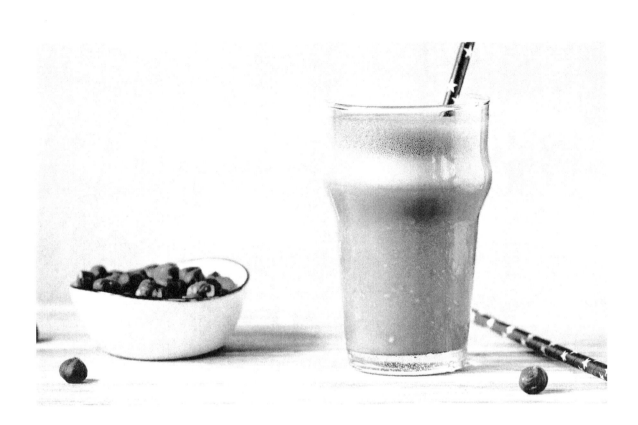

INGREDIENTS

¼ cup unsweetened peanut butter

3 tbsp cocoa powder

1 cup heavy cream (coconut cream for dairy-free or vegan)

1 ½ cup unsweetened almond milk (regular or vanilla)

6 tsp Swerve or sweetener of choice (to taste)

⅛ tsp sea salt (optional)

This is how you make the recipe

1. Combine all ingredients in a blender.

2. Puree until smooth. Adjust sweetener to taste if desired.

3. Serve and enjoy!

FROSTED VANILLA BLACKBERRY LEMONADE

Servings: 1

Nutritional Facts Per Serving:

Net Carbs:	6.95 g	Protein:	8 g
Fat:	2.1 g	Calories:	102 kcal

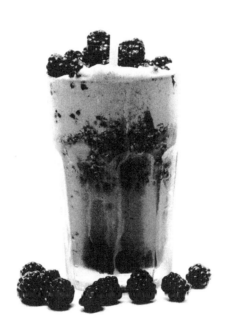

INGREDIENTS

⅔ cup unsweetened almond milk

¼ cup lemon juice

1 tbsp collagen powder

1 tsp Swerve or sweetener of choice

2 pinches sea salt

1 tsp sugar-free vanilla extract

½ tsp glucomannan

½ cup fresh blackberries

3 cups ice cubes

This is how you make the recipe

1. Put lemon juice, almond milk, collagen, Swerve, salt, and vanilla in blender. Turn on low for just a few seconds to mix. While blender is on low, slowly add in glucomannan. Blend on low for 30 seconds and turn off.

2. Add in blackberries and ice cubes, blend on high until completely blended. Notes: Depending on the sweetness of your blackberries, you may need to add a bit more sweetener.

3. Serve and enjoy!

VANILLA ICE CREAM COFFEE SMOOTHIE

Servings: 1

Nutritional Facts Per Serving:

Net Carbs:	2.96 g	Protein:	4.5 g
Fat:	32 g	Calories:	339 kcal

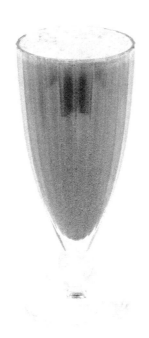

INGREDIENTS

5 cubes coffee frozen in ice cube tray

1 ½ cups unsweetened vanilla almond milk

1 tbsp MCT Oil

1 tbsp chia seeds

2 tbsp heavy whipping cream

1 tsp sugar-free vanilla extract

2 tsp Swerve or sweetener of choice

This is how you make the recipe

1. Freeze coffee in an ice cube tray. (1 ½ cups of coffee will fill a standard ice cube tray.)

2. Add all ingredients icluding 5 cubes of frozen ice cubes of coffee to a blender and blend until smooth.

3. Pour in a glass. Wait 5-8 minutes before serving to allow the chia seeds to thicken the smoothie.

COCONUT MILK STRAWBERRY SMOOTHIE

Servings: 2

Nutritional Facts Per Serving:

Net Carbs:	8.18 g	Protein:	4 g
Fat:	11.5 g	Calories:	153 kcal

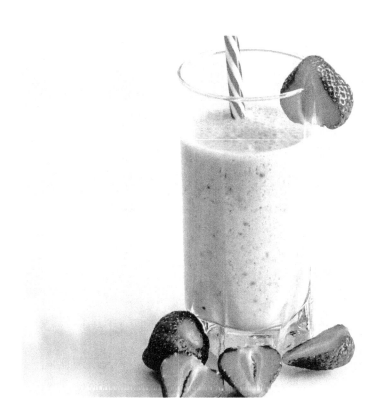

INGREDIENTS

1 cup fresh strawberries

1 cup unsweetened coconut milk

2 tbsp smooth almond butter

2 tbsp Swerve (optional)

This is how you make the recipe

1. Add all ingredients to blender.

2. Blend until smooth.

3. Pour into glass and enjoy!

STRAWBERRY AVOCADO SMOOTHIE

Servings: 2

Nutritional Facts Per Serving:

Net Carbs:	9.3 g	Protein:	4.95 g
Fat:	46.5 g	Calories:	462.5 kcal

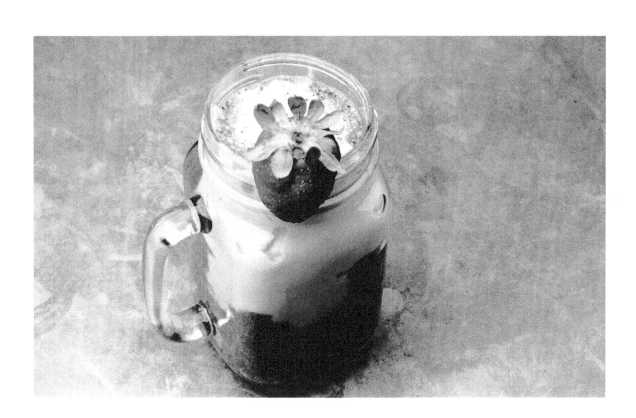

INGREDIENTS

⅔ cup fresh strawberries

1 medium avocado

1 ½ cups unsweetened coconut milk

1 tbsp lime juice

2 tsp Swerve or sweetener of choice

½ cup ice

This is how you make the recipe

1. Add all ingredients into blender and blend until smooth.

2. Serve and enjoy!

CHOCOLATE COVERED MACADAMIA CREEMIE

Servings: 1

Nutritional Facts Per Serving:
Net Carbs: 6.28 g   Protein: 15 g
Fat: 25 g   Calories: 350 kcal

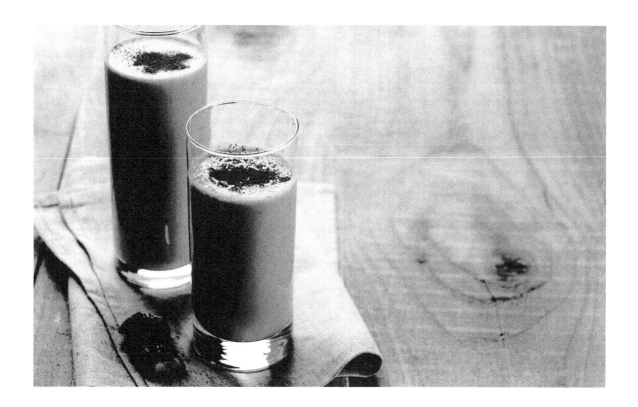

INGREDIENTS

1 cup unsweetened vanilla almond milk

2 tbsp macadamia nuts

1 tsp MCT oil

1 tbsp coconut butter

2 tbsp chia seed

1 tbsp cocoa

1 serving collagen peptides

This is how you make the recipe

1. Blend all ingredients in blender until smooth.
2. Best enjoyed served cold.

MICROGREENS MATCHA SMOOTHIE

Servings: 1

Nutritional Facts Per Serving:

Net Carbs:	4.9 g	Protein:	27 g
Fat:	26 g	Calories:	369 kcal

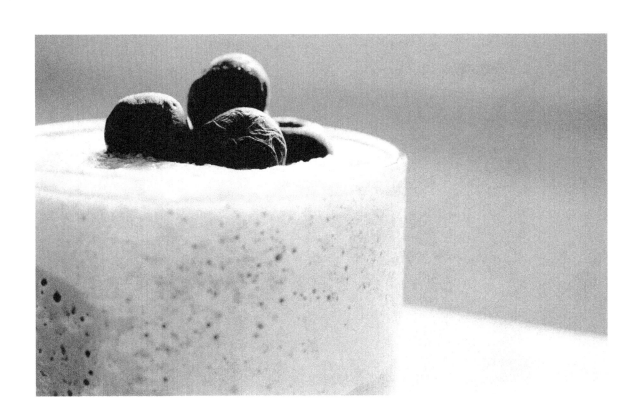

INGREDIENTS

1 scoop microgreens

2 tbsp collagen peptides

1 scoop MCT oil powder

1 tsp matcha powder

¼ cup full-fat coconut milk

¼ cup fresh blueberries

½ cup of ice

1 cup of water

1 tbsp Swerve or sweetener of choice

This is how you make the recipe

1. Combine all of the ingredients, except the collagen in the blender.

2. Blend on high until smooth.

3. Add in the collagen and pulse to combine.

4. Serve and enjoy!

BLUEBERRY GINGER SMOOTHIE

Servings: 2

Nutritional Facts Per Serving:

Net Carbs:	25.7 g	Protein:	8.7 g
Fat:	9.6 g	Calories:	221 kcal

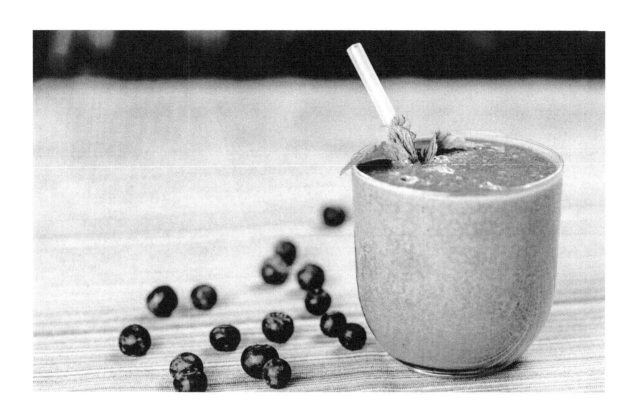

INGREDIENTS

15 fresh blueberries

½ cup coconut yogurt

1 cup unsweetened coconut milk

3 slices of ginger

½ tbsp collagen powder

1 tsp MCT oil

Swerve or sweetener of choice to taste

This is how you make the recipe

1. Blend all ingredients in blender until smooth.
2. Serve and enjoy!

STRAWBERRY & MINT SMOOTHIE

Servings: 2

Nutritional Facts Per Serving:

Net Carbs:	4.9 g	Protein:	2.6 g
Fat:	22.5 g	Calories:	230.5 kcal

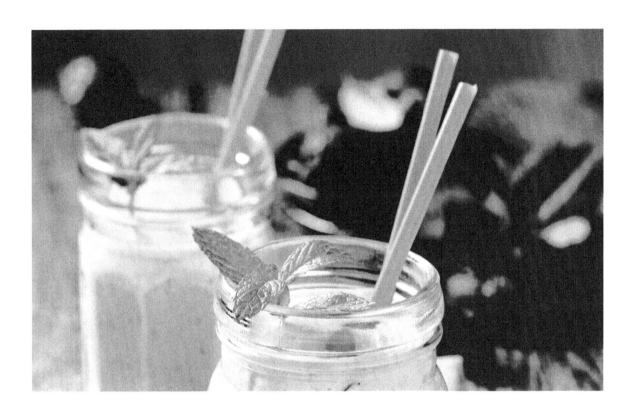

INGREDIENTS

½ cup strawberries

3 tsp scoops cream cheese

Few fresh mint leaves

¼ cup whipping cream

½ cup unsweetened coconut milk

Swerve or sweetener of choice to taste

This is how you make the recipe

1. Blend the strawberries with the cream cheese and mint leaves.

2. Add in the cream, coconut milk and sweetener.

3. Blend together until smooth.

4. Garnish with mint and serve chilled.

SMOOTHIE

Servings: 2

Nutritional Facts Per Serving:
Net Carbs: 7.3 g   Protein: 3.4 g
Fat: 15 g   Calories: 187.5 kcal

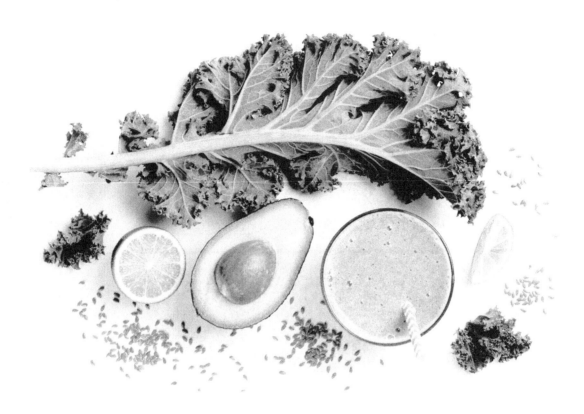

INGREDIENTS

1 cup cold water

1 cup baby spinach

½ cup cilantro

1 inch ginger, peeled

¾ cucumber, peeled

½-1 lemon, peeled

1 cup avocado

This is how you make the recipe

1. Add all ingredients to a blender and blend until smooth.

2. Serve and enjoy!

CHOCOLATE RASPBERRY SPINACH GREEN SMOOTHIE

Servings: 1

Nutritional Facts Per Serving:

Net Carbs:	9.42 g	Protein:	7.5 g
Fat:	44 g	Calories:	467 kcal

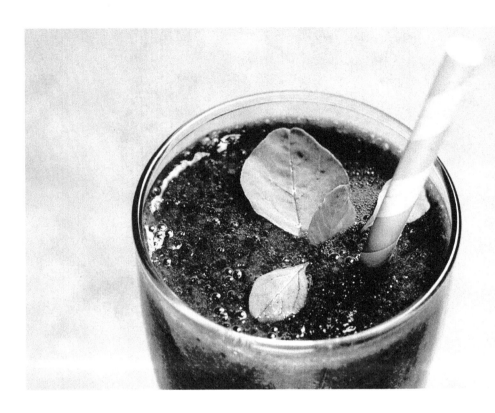

INGREDIENTS

¼ cup fresh raspberries
½ cup spinach
1 tbsp cocoa powder
½ cup heavy cream
½ cup water
1 tbsp Swerve or sweetener of choice
Ice cubes (optional)

This is how you make the recipe

1. Blend all of the ingredients until they combine and become smooth and creamy.

2. Serve and enjoy!

CHOCOLATE BERRY TRUFFLE SMOOTHIE

Servings: 1

Nutritional Facts Per Serving:

Net Carbs:	15.41 g	Protein:	9.2 g
Fat:	42 g	Calories:	507 kcal

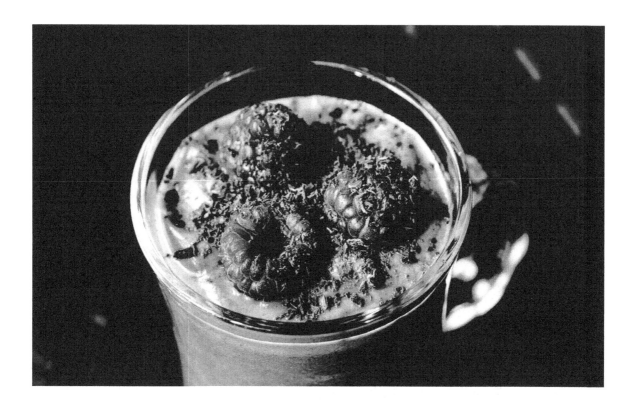

INGREDIENTS

½ medium-sized avocado

2 tbsp raw, unsalted almonds or pecans

1 ½ tbsp unsweetened cocoa powder

1 tbsp Swerve or sweetener of choice

1 pinch sea salt

¾ tsp sugar-free vanilla extract

¼ cup heavy whipping cream

¾ cup fresh mixed berries

Berry bits to garnish (optional)

Cocoa powder to garnish (optional)

This is how you make the recipe

1. Add all ingredients to blender and blend until smooth.

2. Transfer to a glass and add toppings if desired.

3. Serve and enjoy! Note: To make this smoothie not so thick: once the smoothie is blended, pulse in 2 cups of ice cubes until smooth.

SMOOTHIE - PERFECT FOR BREAKFAST

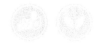

Servings: 2

Nutritional Facts Per Serving:

Net Carbs:	16.8 g	Protein:	14 g
Fat:	102 g	Calories:	1008 kcal

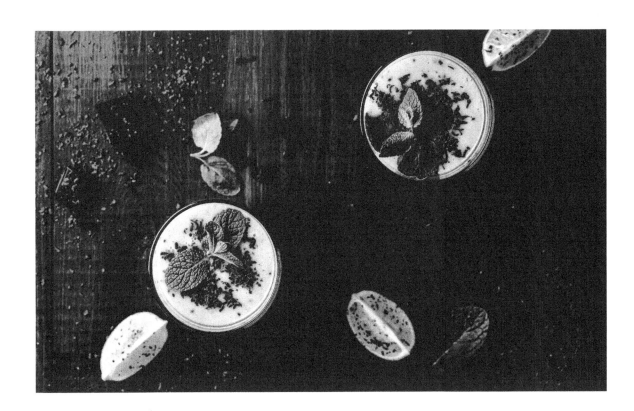

INGREDIENTS

1 ½ cups full-fat coconut milk

⅔ cup ice or cold water

1 tbsp unsweetened peanut butter

2 tsp unsweetened cocoa powder

2 tbsp of Swerve or sweetener of choice

1 medium size avocado

2 ice cubes (optional)

This is how you make the recipe

1. In a blender combine all ingredients and blend until smooth.

2. Serve and enjoy!

CHOCOLATE SMOOTHIE & CHIA SEEDS

Servings: 1

Nutritional Facts Per Serving:
Net Carbs: 23.12 g   Protein: 14 g
Fat: 22 g   Calories: 381 kcal

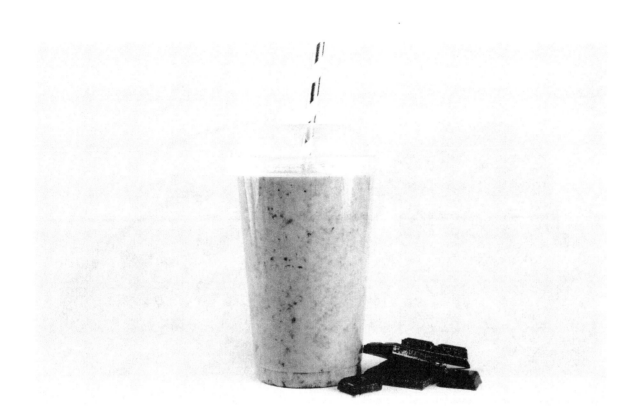

INGREDIENTS

2 tbsp chia seeds

¾ cup water

6 ice cubes

¼ cup whole milk

⅓ cup full-fat Greek yogurt

2 tbsp 100% cocoa dark chocolate

1-2 tsp Swerve or sweetener of choice to taste

This is how you make the recipe

1. Add all ingredients, except the chia seeds into a blender. Blend until smooth.

2. Add the chia seeds and mix into smoothie. If it is too thick, add more water or milk, 1 tbsp at a time.

3. Serve and enjoy!

PEANUT BUTTER AND JELLY SMOOTHIE

Servings: 2

Nutritional Facts Per Serving:

Net Carbs:	11.9 g	Protein:	30 g
Fat:	3.5 g	Calories:	210 kcal

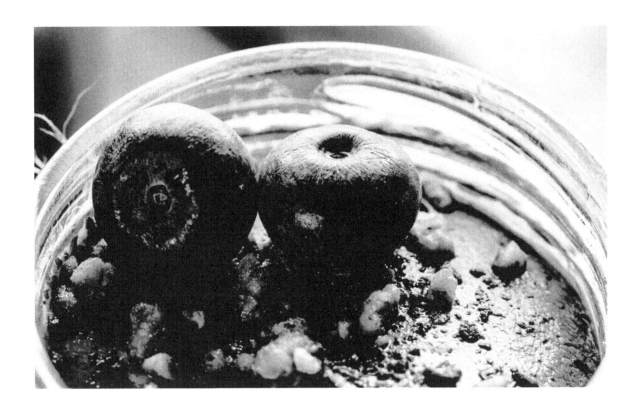

INGREDIENTS

1 cup fresh mixed berries

2 tbsp peanut butter powder

1 scoop dairy free vanilla protein powder

1 ½ cups dairy free almond milk

1 scoop keto friendly protein powder of choice

This is how you make the recipe

1. Combine all ingredients in a blender and pulse until smooth and creamy.

2. Serve and enjoy!

BLUEBERRY SMOOTHIE

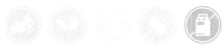

Servings: 2

Nutritional Facts Per Serving:

Net Carbs:	9.75 g	Protein:	4.2 g
Fat:	42.5 g	Calories:	413.5 kcal

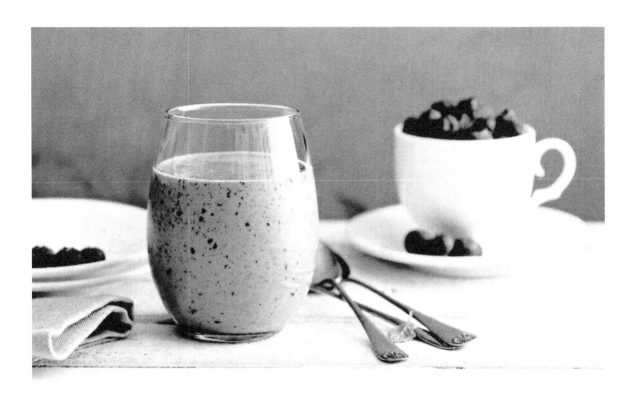

INGREDIENTS

1 ½ cups unsweetened coconut milk

½ cup fresh blueberries

1 tbsp lemon juice

½ tsp sugar-free vanilla extract

This is how you make the recipe

1. Place all ingredients in a blender and mix until smooth. Using canned coconut milk makes a creamier, more satisfying smoothie.

2. Taste, and add more lemon juice if desired.

3. Serve and enjoy!

ACAI ALMOND BUTTER SMOOTHIE

Servings: 1

Nutritional Facts Per Serving:

Net Carbs:	4.21 g	Protein:	24 g
Fat:	36 g	Calories:	451 kcal

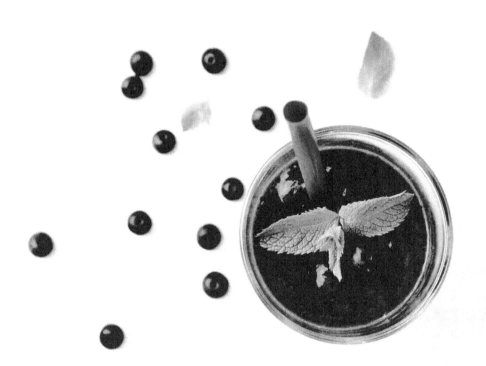

INGREDIENTS

1 100g pack unsweetened Acai Puree

¾ cup unsweetened almond milk

¼ avocado

3 tbsp collagen or protein powder

1 tbsp coconut oil or MCT oil powder

1 tbsp unsweetened almond butter

½ tsp sugar-free vanilla extract

1 tsp Swerve (optional)

This is how you make the recipe

1. If you are using individualized 100 gram packs of acai puree, run the pack under lukewarm water for a few seconds until you are able to break up the puree into smaller pieces. Open the pack and put the contents into the blender.

2. Place the remaining ingredients in the blender and blend until smooth. Add more water or ice cubes as needed.

3. Serve and enjoy!

CINNAMON ALMOND BUTTER BREAKFAST SHAKE

Servings: 1

Nutritional Facts Per Serving:

Net Carbs:	4 g	Protein:	17 g
Fat:	27 g	Calories:	339 kcal

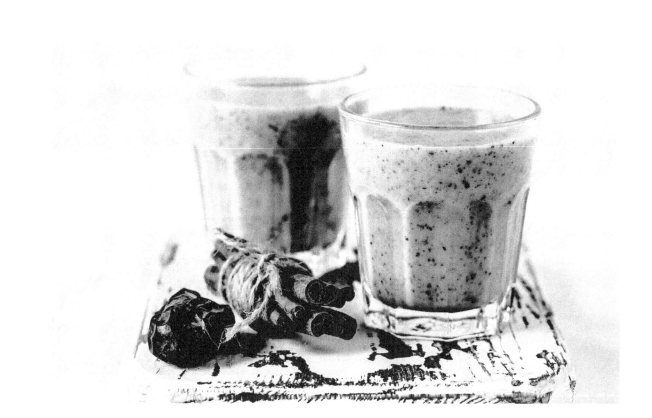

INGREDIENTS

1 ½ cups unsweetened nut milk

1 scoop collagen peptides

2 tbsp almond butter

2 tbsp golden flax meal

½ tsp cinnamon

2 tsp Swerve or sweetener of choice

⅛ tsp almond extract

⅛ tsp sea salt

6 ice cubes

This is how you make the recipe

1. Add all the ingredients to a blender and combine for 30 seconds or until you get a smooth consistency.

2. Serve and enjoy!

MATCHA GREEN TEA SMOOTHIE

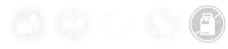

Servings: 1

Nutritional Facts Per Serving:

Net Carbs:	2.5 g	Protein:	5.4 g
Fat:	7 g	Calories:	108 kcal

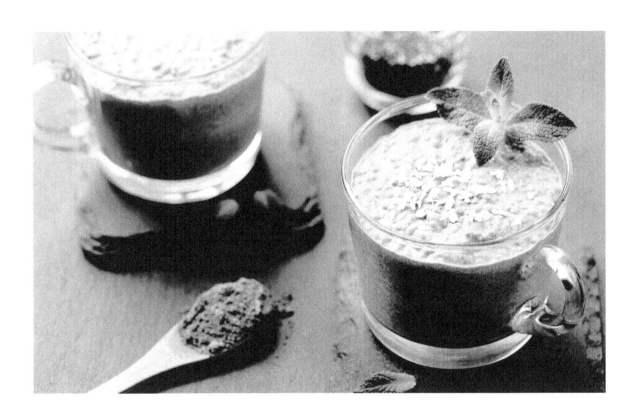

INGREDIENTS

¾ cup unsweetened almond milk or coconut milk

1 tbsp chia seeds

1 tsp matcha green tea powder

¼ tsp lemon juice

1 tsp Swerve or sweetener of choice

2 tbsp plain Greek yogurt or use coconut cream for dairy free

¼ tsp glucomannan or xanthan gum

¼ cup crushed ice (optional)

This is how you make the recipe

1. Combine all ingredients with blender until smooth.

2. Serve and enjoy!

MINUTE MOCHA SMOOTHIE

Servings: 3

Nutritional Facts Per Serving:

Net Carbs:	4.3 g	Protein:	3.2 g
Fat:	16.7 g	Calories:	189.3 kcal

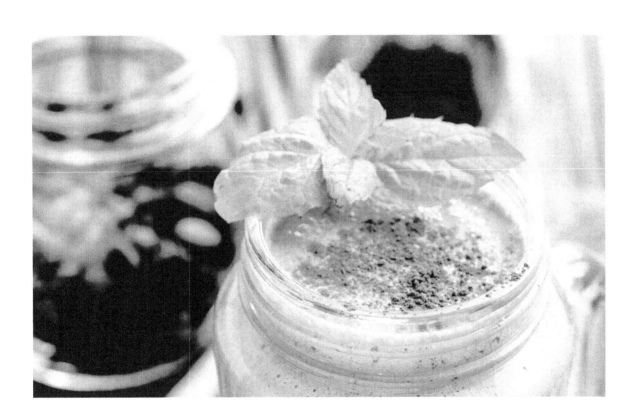

INGREDIENTS

½ cup coconut milk (the thick stuff from a can)

1 ½ cup unsweetened almond milk

1 tsp sugar-free vanilla extract

3 tbsp Swerve or sweetener of choice

2 tsp instant coffee crystals, regular or decaffeinated

3 tbsp unsweetened cocoa powder

1 avocado cut in half with pit removed

This is how you make the recipe

1. Place coconut milk, almond milk, sugar-free vanilla extract, sweetener, coffee crystals, and cocoa powder into a blender. Blend until smooth.

2. Scoop the avocado into the mixture. Blend until smooth.

3. Serve and enjoy!

STRAWBERRY AVOCADO SMOOTHIE WITH ALMOND MILK - 4 INGREDIENTS

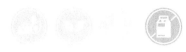

Servings: 5

Nutritional Facts Per Serving:

Net Carbs:	7.98 g	Protein:	1.28 g
Fat:	5 g	Calories:	90.2 kcal

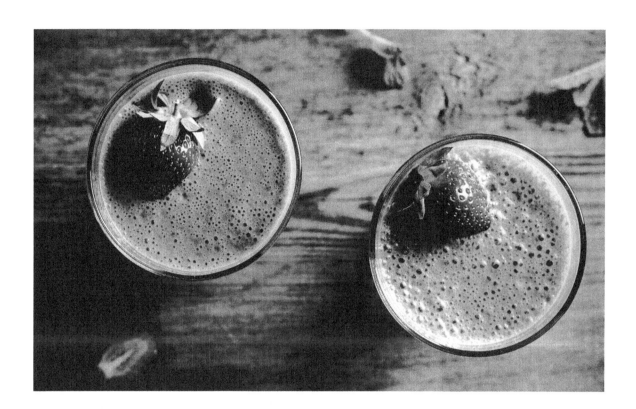

INGREDIENTS

2 cups fresh strawberries

1 ½ cups unsweetened almond milk (regular or vanilla)

1 large avocado

¼ cup Swerve or sweetener of choice (adjust amount to taste)

This is how you make the recipe

1. Puree all ingredients in a blender, until smooth.

2. Adjust sweetener to taste as needed. Note: For a richer, creamier smoothie, swap out half of the almond milk with coconut cream, or heavy cream if you're not dairy-free.

3. Serve and enjoy!

AVOCADO SMOOTHIE WITH COCONUT MILK, GINGER AND TURMERIC

Servings: 2

Nutritional Facts Per Serving:

Net Carbs:	4.7 g	Protein:	2.65 g
Fat:	23.5 g	Calories:	234.5 kcal

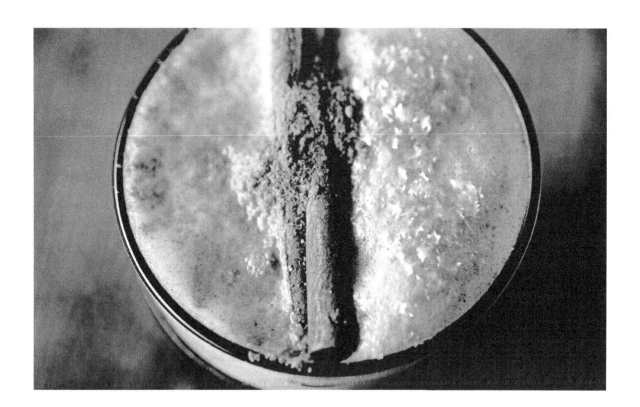

INGREDIENTS

½ avocado

¾ cup unsweetened coconut milk

¼ cup unsweetened almond milk

1 tsp fresh grated ginger (about ½ inch piece)

½ tsp turmeric

1 tsp lemon or lime juice (more to taste)

1 cup crushed ice

Swerve or sweetener of choice to taste

This is how you make the recipe

1. Add the first 6 ingredients to a blender and blend on low-speed until smooth.

2. Add crushed ice and sweetener. Blend on high until smooth.

3. Taste and adjust sweetness and tartness per your taste buds.

4. Serve and enjoy!

AVOCADO MINT GREEN SMOOTHIE

Servings: 1

Nutritional Facts Per Serving:

Net Carbs:	13.5 g	Protein:	5.6 g
Fat:	48 g	Calories:	491 kcal

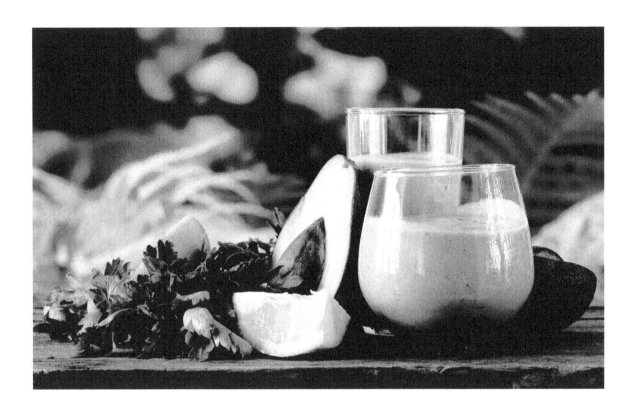

INGREDIENTS

½ avocado

¾ cup full-fat coconut milk

½ cup unsweetened almond milk

Swerve or sweetener of choice to taste

5-6 large mint leaves

3 sprigs of cilantro

1 squeeze of lime juice

¼ tsp sugar-free vanilla extract

1 cup crushed ice

This is how you make the recipe

1. Place all of the ingredients in blender, blend until smooth. Taste to adjust sweetness and tartness.

2. Serve and enjoy!

BLUEBERRY COCONUT YOGURT SMOOTHIE

Servings: 2

Nutritional Facts Per Serving:

Net Carbs:	4.2 g	Protein:	2.35 g
Fat:	24 g	Calories:	229.5 kcal

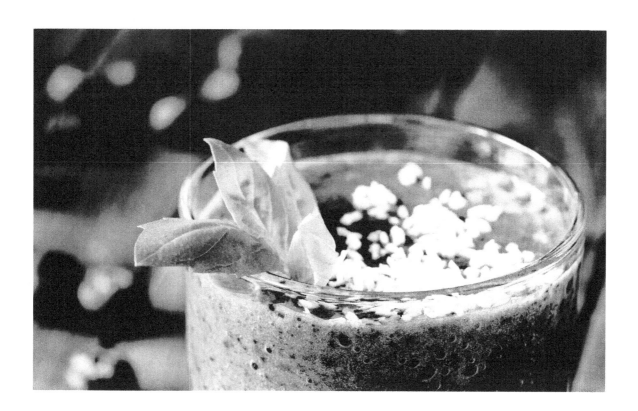

INGREDIENTS

10 fresh blueberries

1 cup coconut milk

½ tsp sugar-free vanilla extract

Swerve or sweetener of choice to taste

This is how you make the recipe

1. Place all of the ingredients in blender, blend until smooth.

2. Serve and enjoy!

RASPBERRY AVOCADO SMOOTHIE

Servings: 2

Nutritional Facts Per Serving:

Net Carbs:	19.8 g	Protein:	1.95 g
Fat:	10.5 g	Calories:	191.5 kcal

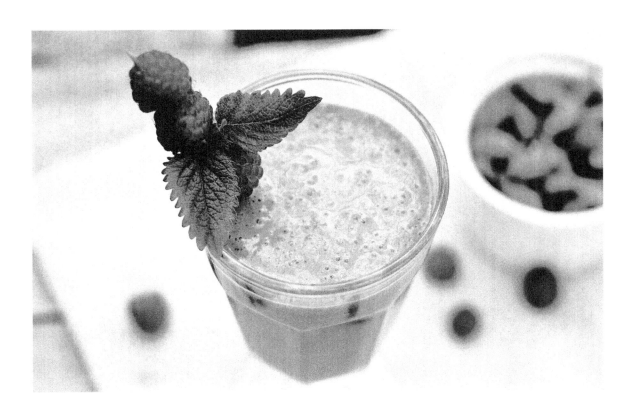

INGREDIENTS

1 avocado, peeled and pit removed

1 ⅓ cup water

3 tbsp lemon juice

2 tbsp Swerve or sweetener of choice

½ cup fresh raspberries

This is how you make the recipe

1. Add all ingredients to blender.

2. Blend until smooth.

3. Pour into two tall glasses and enjoy with a straw!

CHIA PUMPKIN SMOOTHIE

Servings: 1

Nutritional Facts Per Serving:

Net Carbs:	10.7 g	Protein:	6.6 g
Fat:	71 g	Calories:	713 kcal

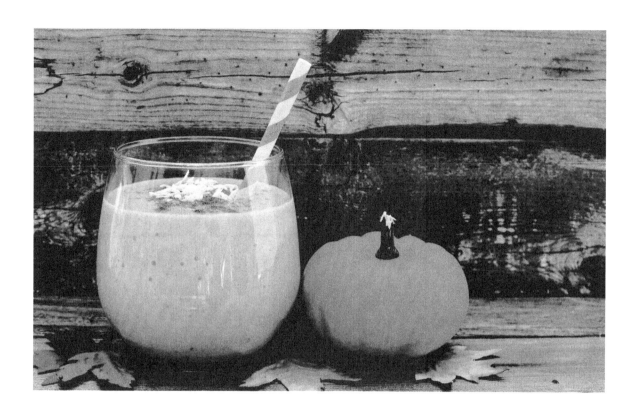

INGREDIENTS

¾ cup full-fat coconut milk

3 tbsp pumpkin puree

1 tbsp MCT oil (optional)

1 tsp loose chia tea

1 tsp sugar-free vanilla extract

½ tsp pumpkin pie spice

½ avocado

This is how you make the recipe

1. Add all ingredients but avocado to the blender and blend until smooth.

2. Add the avocado and blend until broken apart.

3. Serve and enjoy with a sprinkle of pumpkin spice on top, if you'd like.

TURMERIC SMOOTHIE

Servings: 1

Nutritional Facts Per Serving:

Net Carbs:	12.7 g	Protein:	8 g
Fat:	61 g	Calories:	629 kcal

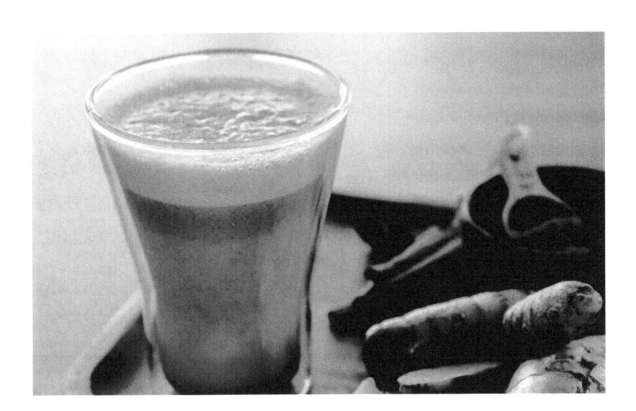

INGREDIENTS

1 cup full-fat coconut milk

1 cup unsweetened almond milk

1 Swerve or sweetener of choice

1 tbsp ground turmeric

1 tsp ground cinnamon

1 tsp ground ginger

1 tbsp MCT oil or use coconut oil

1 tbsp chia seeds (to garnish)

½ cup ice cubes

This is how you make the recipe

1. Combine all the ingredients except the chia seeds in a blender, add some ice and blend until smooth .

2. Sprinkle chia seeds on top and enjoy!

CHOCOLATE MINT AVOCADO SMOOTHIE

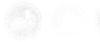

Servings: 1

Nutritional Facts Per Serving:

Net Carbs:	8.9 g	Protein:	28 g
Fat:	51 g	Calories:	599 kcal

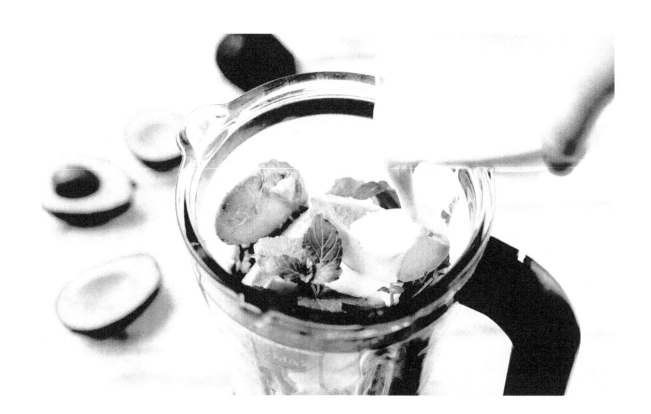

INGREDIENTS

½ cup coconut milk

1 cup water

½ cup ice cubes

2 scoops chocolate collagen protein

½ avocado

4 mint leaves

1 tbsp crushed cacao butter

2 tbsp shredded coconut

This is how you make the recipe

1. Add all ingredients excluding the collagen protein and shredded coconut to a blender.

2. Blend for 45 seconds on high.

3. Add collagen protein and blend for 5 seconds on low.

4. Top with coconut flakes and enjoy!

CINNAMON CHOCOLATE BREAKFAST SMOOTHIE

Servings: 1

Nutritional Facts Per Serving:

Net Carbs:	8.2 g	Protein:	5.5 g
Fat:	54 g	Calories:	531 kcal

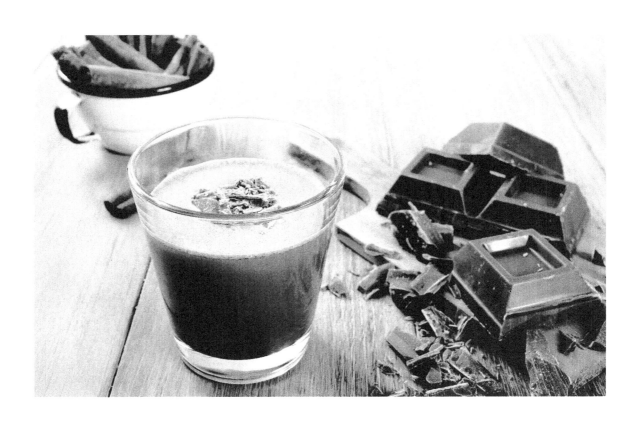

INGREDIENTS

¾ cup coconut milk
½ avocado
2 tsp unsweetened cacao powder
1 tsp cinnamon powder
¼ tsp sugar-free vanilla extract
Swerve or sweetener of choice to taste
½ tsp MCT oil or 1 tsp coconut oil (optional)

This is how you make the recipe

1. Blend all the ingredients together well.
2. Serve and enjoy!

CHOCOLATE COCONUT SMOOTHIE BOWL

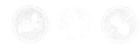

Servings: 1

Nutritional Facts Per Serving:

Net Carbs:	8.8 g	Protein:	27 g
Fat:	37 g	Calories:	465 kcal

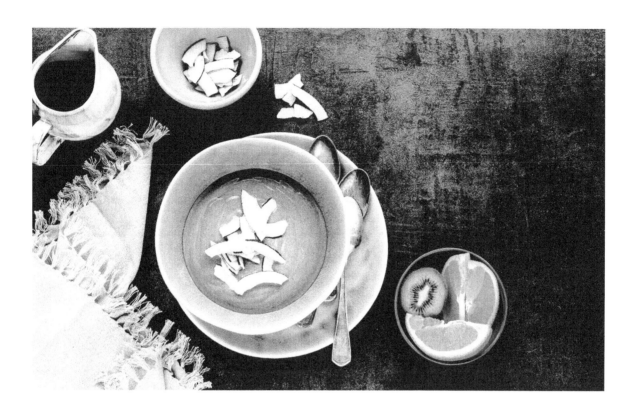

INGREDIENTS

¾ cup full-fat coconut milk

2 tbsp unsweetened cocoa powder

1 tbsp Swerve or sweetener of choice

½ cup ice cubes

2 scoops collagen protein

This is how you make the recipe

1. Place all of the ingredients except the collagen in a blender and blend well.

2. Add the collagen and gently pulse until blended.

3. Place in a bowl and add optional garnishes and enjoy!

GREEN BREAKFAST SMOOTHIE

Servings: 1

Nutritional Facts Per Serving:

Net Carbs:	15.75 g	Protein:	11 g
Fat:	31 g	Calories:	393 kcal

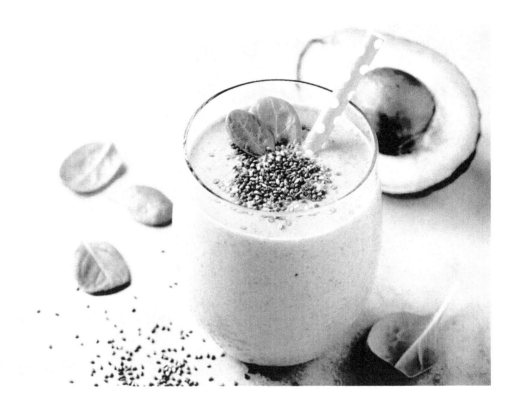

INGREDIENTS

1 ½ cups unsweetened almond milk

1 oz spinach

⅓ cup cucumber

⅓ cup celery

⅓ cup avocado

1 tbsp coconut oil

1 tbsp Swerve or sweetener of choice

1 egg

½ tsp chia seeds (to garnish)

1 tsp matcha powder (optional)

This is how you make the recipe

1. Into a blender, add your almond milk and spinach. Blend for a second to break down the spinach to make room for the rest of the ingredients.

2. Add in the rest of your ingredients and blend for about a minute until creamy.

3. You can add a teaspoon of matcha powder for added benefits and a kick of caffeine.

4. Pour it into a glass and garnish with chia seeds. Enjoy!

FROZEN BERRY SHAKE

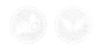

Servings: 1

Nutritional Facts Per Serving:

Net Carbs:	11.84 g	Protein:	3.5 g
Fat:	39 g	Calories:	404 kcal

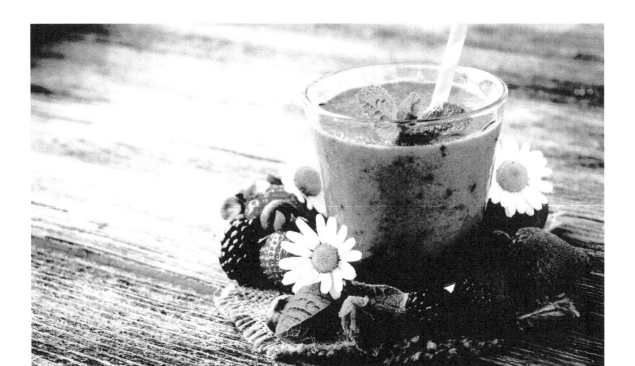

INGREDIENTS

⅓ cup creamed coconut milk or heavy whipping cream

½ cup water or almond milk

½ cup mixed berries

1 tbsp MCT oil or coconut oil

½ cup ice cubes

Optionally add:

1 tbsp Swerve or sweetener of choice

½ tsp sugar-free vanilla extract

Whipped cream or coconut milk on top

This is how you make the recipe

1. To "cream" the coconut milk, simply place the can in the fridge overnight. Next day, open, spoon out the solidified coconut milk and discard the liquids. Do not shake before opening the can. Place the creamed coconut milk, berries, water or almond milk and ice into a blender.

2. Add MCT oil and Swerve (optional).

3. Pulse until smooth and serve immediately. You can top with whipped cream or coconut milk (optional).

CLEAN & GREEN SMOOTHIE

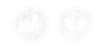

Servings: 1

Nutritional Facts Per Serving:

Net Carbs:	6 g	Protein:	3.1 g
Fat:	24 g	Calories:	267 kcal

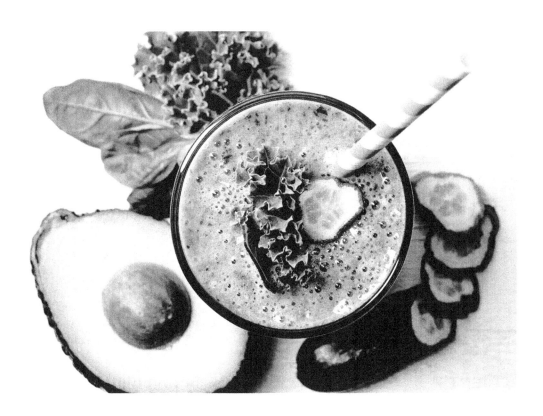

INGREDIENTS

1 cup water

½ avocado

1 tbsp MCT oil

½ cucumber

1 large handful dark leafy greens

1–2 leaves dandelion

2 tbsp parsley

Juice from 1 lemon

¼ tsp turmeric powder

This is how you make the recipe

1. Blend all ingredients in a high-speed blender until smooth.

2. Best enjoyed cold.

BLUEBERRY GALAXY SMOOTHIE

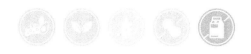

Servings: 1

Nutritional Facts Per Serving:
Net Carbs: 12.36 g   Protein: 30 g
Fat: 53 g   Calories: 631 kcal

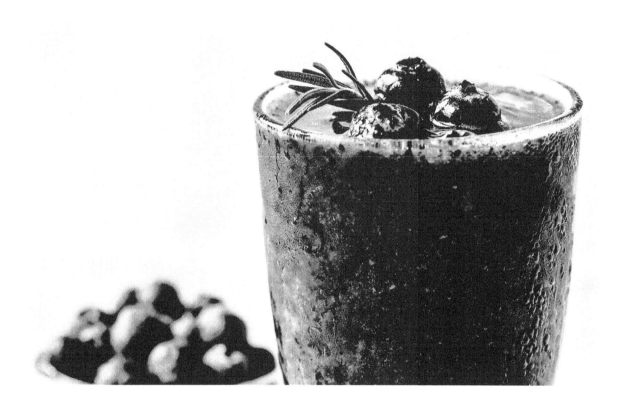

INGREDIENTS

1 cup coconut milk

¼ cup blueberries

1 tsp sugar-free vanilla extract

1 tsp MCT oil

1 scoop protein powder (optional)

This is how you make the recipe

1. Put all the ingredients into a mixer, and blend until smooth. Note: If you would like a swirl, add a tablespoon of some full-fat yogurt after the smoothie is in a glass, and swirl it around, touching the sides.

2. Serve and enjoy!

RASPBERRY LEMONADE SMOOTHIE

Servings: 4

Nutritional Facts Per Serving:

Net Carbs:	7.24 g	Protein:	7.5 g
Fat:	5.5 g	Calories:	119.25 kcal

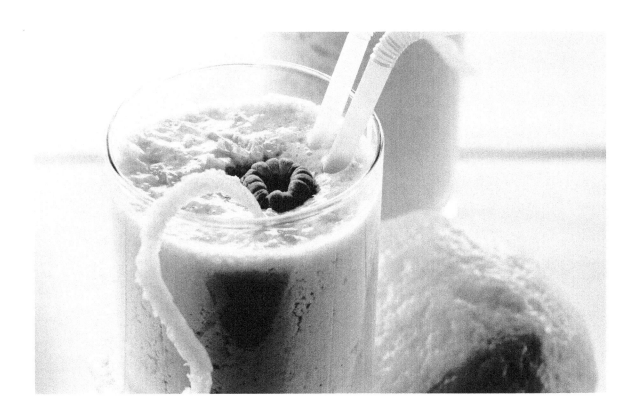

INGREDIENTS

1 cup fresh raspberries

1 cup Greek yogurt

⅓ cup freshly squeezed lemon juice

⅓ cup water

¼ cup Swerve or sweetener of choice

¼ cup cream cheese

1 tsp lemon zest

2 cups ice cubes

This is how you make the recipe

1. In a blender, combine raspberries, yogurt, lemon juice, water, sweetener, cream cheese, lemon zest, and ice. Blend until smooth. Adjust sweetener to taste.

2. Divide between 4 glasses and enjoy!

COLD BREW PROTEIN SHAKE SMOOTHIE

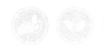

Servings: 1

Nutritional Facts Per Serving:

Net Carbs:	2.46 g	Protein:	0.6 g
Fat:	0.9 g	Calories:	21 kcal

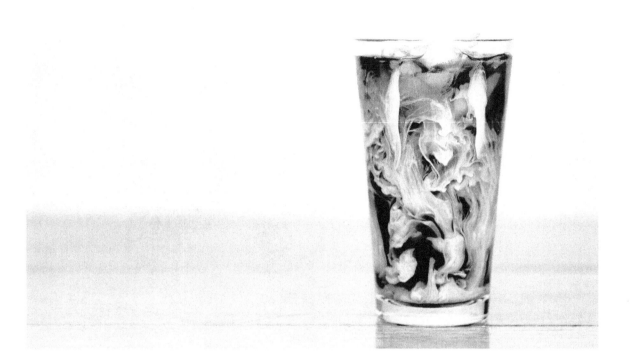

1 cup cold brew coffee

⅓ cup almond milk or heavy cream

½ cup ice cubes

This is how you make the recipe

1. Combine all ingredients in a milk frother or a shaker bottle. Mix until well combined.

2. Serve and enjoy!

RED VELVET SMOOTHIE

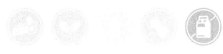

Servings: 2

Nutritional Facts Per Serving:

Net Carbs: 9.45 g   Protein: 6 g

Fat: 54 g   Calories: 523.5 kcal

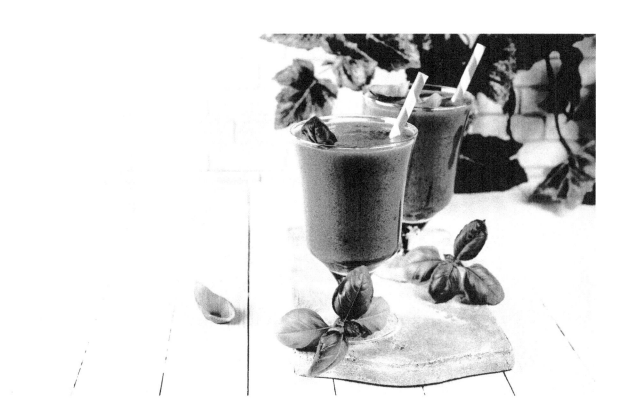

INGREDIENTS

2 cups coconut milk or almond milk

2 cups ice cubes

½ avocado

½ small beet

3 tbsp unsweetened cocoa powder

¼ tsp sugar-free vanilla extract

2 tbsp Swerve or sweetener of choice

This is how you make the recipe

1. Put all the ingredients in a blender and mix until completely smooth.

2. Adjust sweetness to taste. Note: If you have a weak blender, boil your beets first.

3. Serve and enjoy!

ANTI-INFLAMMATORY GREEN SMOOTHIE

Servings: 1-2

Nutritional Facts Per Serving:
Net Carbs: 5 g   Protein: 0.9 g
Fat: 0.2 g   Calories: 24.5 kcal

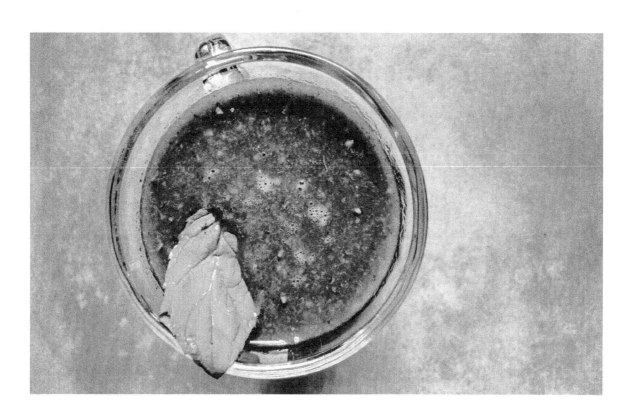

INGREDIENTS

1 cup ice cubes

½ cucumber

1 celery stalk

1 romaine lettuce leaf

1 whole lime, peeled

1 tsp green powder

1 tsp ginger powder

Pinch turmeric powder

1 cup water

This is how you make the recipe

1. Place all ingredients in a blender, blend until smooth.

2. Serve and enjoy!

COCONUT RASPBERRY VANILLA SMOOTHIE

Servings: 2

Nutritional Facts Per Serving:

Net Carbs:	3.4 g	Protein:	1.2 g
Fat:	8 g	Calories:	92.5 kcal

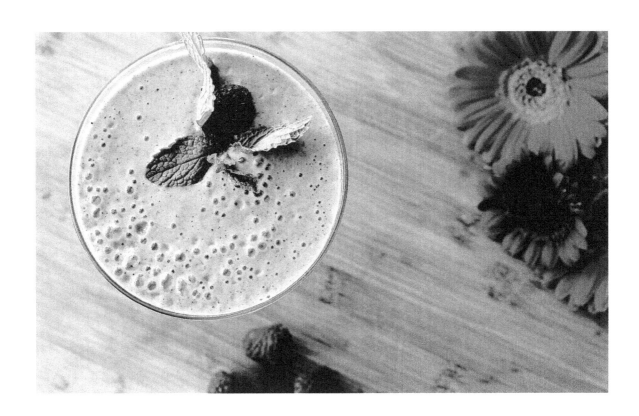

INGREDIENTS

⅓ cup full-fat coconut milk

¼ cup water

⅛ tsp pure vanilla powder

Pinch of finely ground sea salt

⅓ cup fresh raspberries

8 ice cubes

This is how you make the recipe

1. Combine all ingredients in a blender, blend until smooth.

2. Serve and enjoy!

STRAWBERRY COCONUT SMOOTHIE

Servings: 1

Nutritional Facts Per Serving:

Net Carbs:	16.5 g	Protein:	5.8 g
Fat:	25 g	Calories:	349 kcal

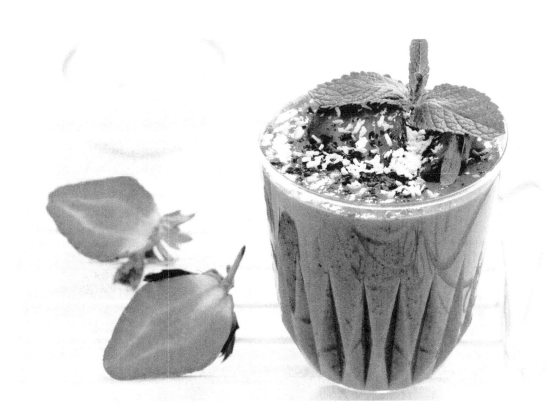

INGREDIENTS

1 cup nut milk

5-6 fresh strawberries

2 tbsp coconut manna

1 tbsp chia seed

Shredded coconut (for garnish)

This is how you make the recipe

1. Combine nut milk, frozen strawberries, coconut manna, chia seed in blender.

2. Blend on high until ingredients are well combined.

3. Serve, top with optional shredded coconut and enjoy!

"SLEEP IN" SMOOTHIE

Servings: 2

Nutritional Facts Per Serving:

Net Carbs:	12 g	Protein:	5.5 g
Fat:	5.5 g	Calories:	123.5 kcal

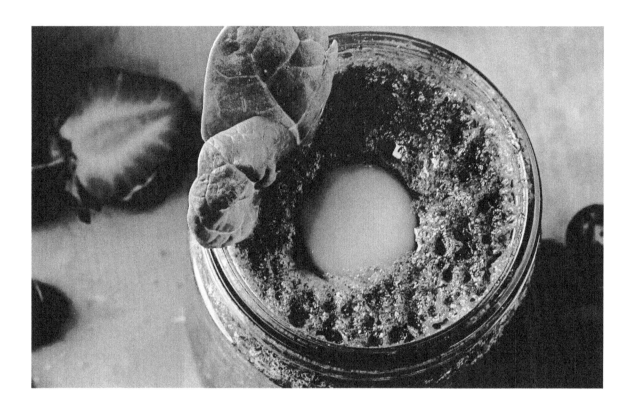

INGREDIENTS

1 raw egg

¼ cup of kombucha (water/ coconut milk or almond milk)

1 cup mixed berries

2 cups spinach

¼ avocado

This is how you make the recipe

1. Combine all ingredients in a blender, blend until smooth.

2. Serve and enjoy!

CHOCOLATE GREEN SMOOTHIE

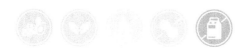

Servings: 2

Nutritional Facts Per Serving:

Net Carbs:	12.4 g	Protein:	4.3 g
Fat:	27 g	Calories:	330 kcal

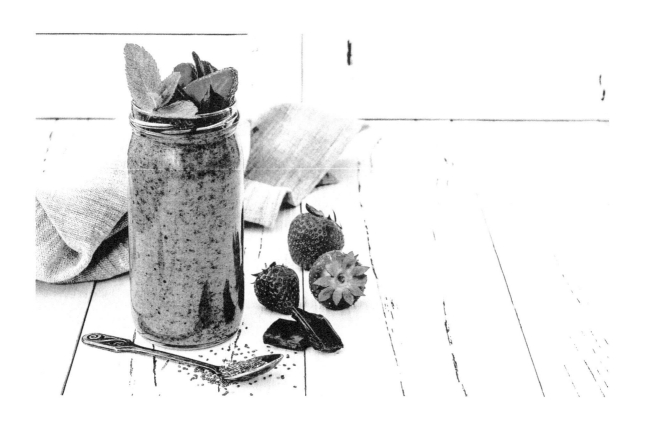

INGREDIENTS

½ cup fresh berries

1 cup unsweetened coconut cream

½ cup spinach, chopped

3 tbsp unsweetened cocoa powder

1 tbsp Swerve or sweetener of choice

This is how you make the recipe

1. Put everything in a blender and blend until smooth.

2. Serve and enjoy!

HYDRATING MATCHA SMOOTHIE

Servings: 2

Nutritional Facts Per Serving:

Net Carbs:	5.5 g	Protein:	7.5 g
Fat:	21.5 g	Calories:	253.5 kcal

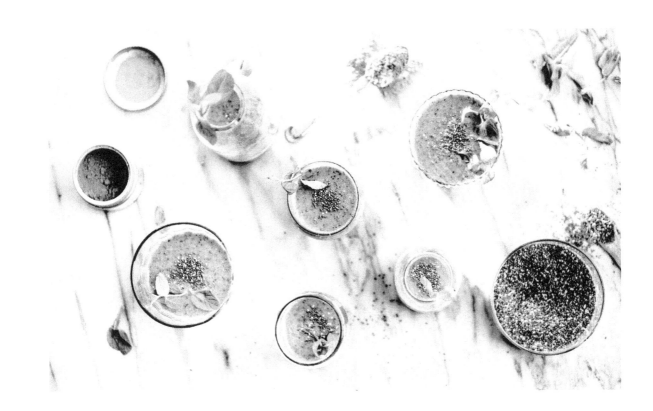

INGREDIENTS

1 cup cauliflower florets, steamed

2 scoops collagen powder

1 tsp matcha

1 tsp sugar-free vanilla extract

5 drops Stevia (optional)

½ cup water

½ cup coconut or nut milk

1 tbsp chia seeds

2 tbsp cocoa powder

1 tbsp coconut oil

Shredded coconut (optional)

This is how you make the recipe

1. Combine the cauliflower, coconut milk, water, Swerve, vanilla, collagen and matcha in your blender. Blend on high until thick and smooth, the chia seeds should be pulverized.

2. In a microwave safe bowl combine the coconut oil and cocoa powder, microwave for 20-30 seconds, then stir until a thin chocolate sauce forms.

3. Pour smoothie into a bowl and drizzle chocolate sauce over it, it will harden when it touches the cold smoothie, like magic shell!

4. Sprinkle with shredded coconut and enjoy!

PROBIOTIC GREEN SMOOTHIE

Servings: 1

Nutritional Facts Per Serving:

Net Carbs:	14.9 g	Protein:	17 g
Fat:	39 g	Calories:	497 kcal

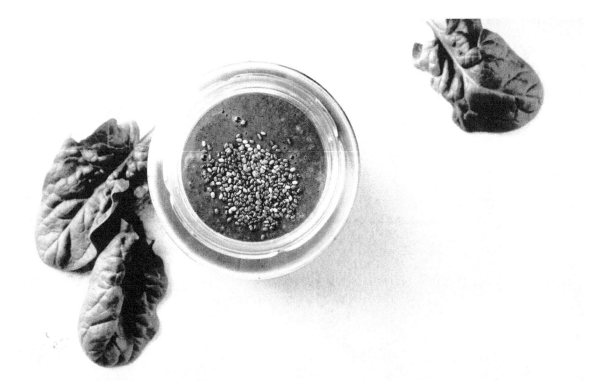

INGREDIENTS

1 handful baby spinach

1 cup kombucha tea

½ cup coconut milk

½ avocado

½ cup fresh mixed berries

1 tbsp grass-fed collagen

1 tbsp chia seeds

This is how you make the recipe

1. Combine all ingredients except for the chia seeds in a blender.

2. Once the ingredients are smooth, add in the chia seeds and do a couple quick pulses to combine.

3. Serve and enjoy!

SUMMER MORNING GREEN SMOOTHIE

Servings: 2

Nutritional Facts Per Serving:

| Net Carbs: | 17.8 g | Protein: | 7.5 g |
| Fat: | 12 g | Calories: | 219.5 kcal |

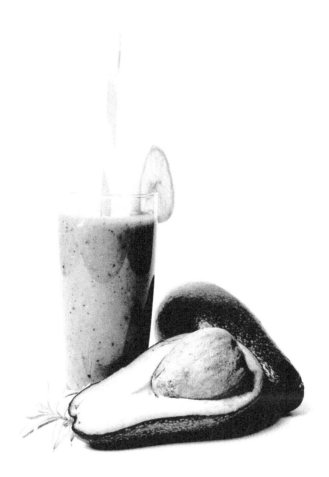

INGREDIENTS

½ large seedless cucumber

½ lemon, most seeds removed

1 avocado

4 cups fresh kale

1 ½ cups water

This is how you make the recipe

1. Add cucumber, lemon, and avocado into your blender.

2. Pack the rest of the container with your kale, and then add water. Pulse until smooth.

3. Serve and enjoy!

REFRESHING CUCUMBER CELERY LIME SMOOTHIE

Servings: 2

Nutritional Facts Per Serving:

Net Carbs:	5.6 g	Protein:	1.3 g
Fat:	0.3 g	Calories:	30.5 kcal

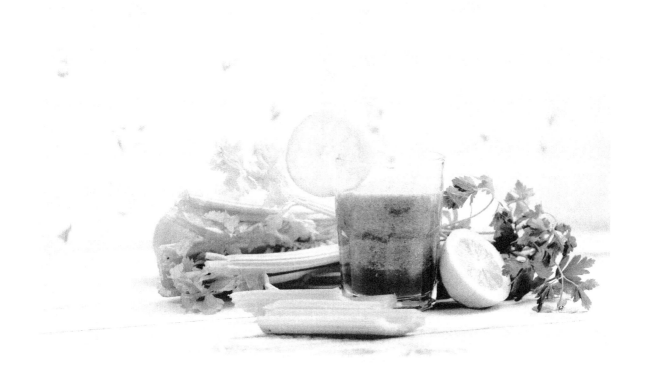

INGREDIENTS

4 stalks celery, chopped large chunks
1 small cucumber, peeled and chopped, seeds removed
½ lime juice
½ cup water
½ cup ice cubes

This is how you make the recipe

1. Place everything into a blender and blend until smooth. (If you want it to be a juice, then just strain the smoothie.)

2. Serve and enjoy!

RED SMOOTHIE

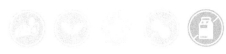

Servings: 2

Nutritional Facts Per Serving:

Net Carbs:	32.9 g	Protein:	10 g
Fat:	50.5 g	Calories:	647 kcal

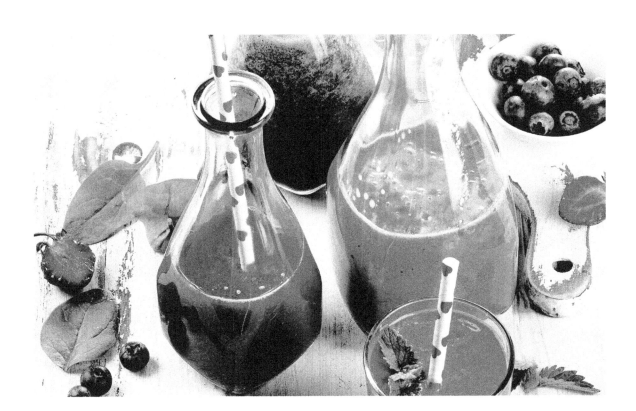

INGREDIENTS

2 cups fresh strawberries

2 cups fresh raspberries, plus more for garnish (optional)

2 cups fresh blackberries

2 cups coconut milk

1 cup baby spinach

Unsweetened shaved coconut to garnish (optional)

This is how you make the recipe

1. In a blender, combine all ingredients (except for coconut). Blend until smooth.

2. Divide between cups and top with raspberries and coconut as garnish (optional).

MINTY COOL SMOOTHIE

Servings: 1

Nutritional Facts Per Serving:
Net Carbs: 5.58 g   Protein: 8.7 g
Fat: 27 g   Calories: 287 kcal

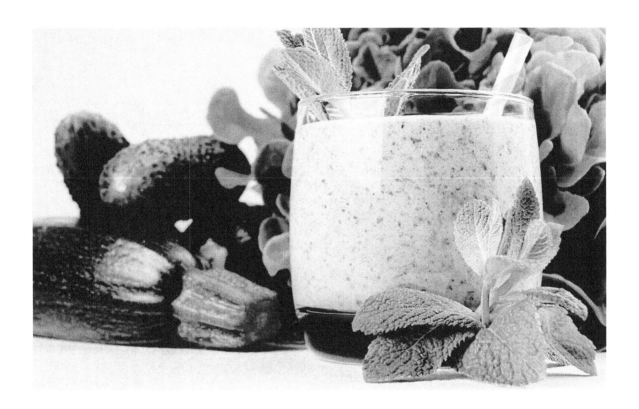

INGREDIENTS

½ cup cucumber (peeled and seeded)

1 tbsp fresh mint

½ cup unsweetened coconut milk

1 cup water

1 cup fresh spinach

3-4 ice cubes

1 scoop unsweetened protein powder

This is how you make the recipe

1. Combine all ingredients and blend together in blender until smooth.

2. Serve and enjoy!

CHOCOLATE SMOOTHIE

   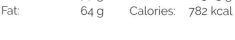

Servings: 2

Nutritional Facts Per Serving:

Net Carbs:	17.7 g	Protein:	32.5 g
Fat:	64 g	Calories:	782 kcal

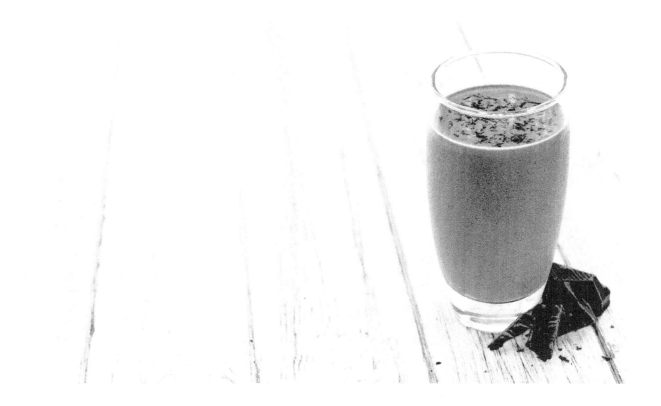

INGREDIENTS

1 can full-fat coconut milk
¼ cup egg white protein powder
2 tbsp ground chia seeds
½ tsp Swerve or sweetener of
choice
½ cup chopped 85% dark
chocolate
2-3 cups ice

This is how you make the recipe

1. In a blender combine coconut milk, protein powder, chia, and sweetener, blend until smooth.

2. Blend in chocolate until smooth.

3. Blend in ice cubes until mixture is well combined.

4. Serve and enjoy!

GREEN SMOOTHIE

Servings: 1

Nutritional Facts Per Serving:

Net Carbs:	6.3 g	Protein:	10 g
Fat:	19 g	Calories:	248 kcal

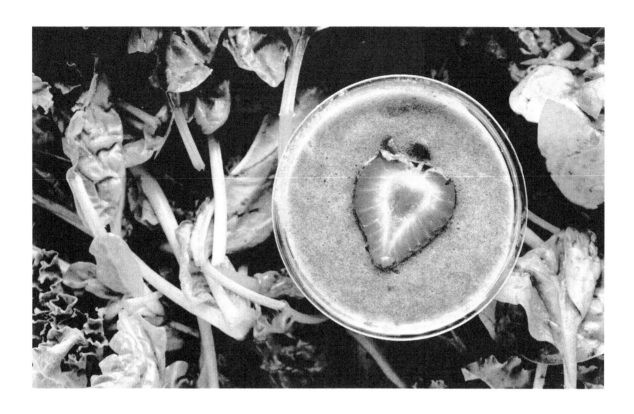

INGREDIENTS

3 fresh strawberries

½ cup fresh spinach or kale

1 tsp chia seeds

2 tbsp unsweetened almond butter

1 tbsp Swerve or sweetener of choice

1 cup water or almond milk

This is how you make the recipe

1. Add all to a blender and blend until smooth.

2. Serve and enjoy!

AVOCADO SMOOTHIE

Servings: 1

Nutritional Facts Per Serving:

Net Carbs:	8.56 g	Protein:	32 g
Fat:	51 g	Calories:	619 kcal

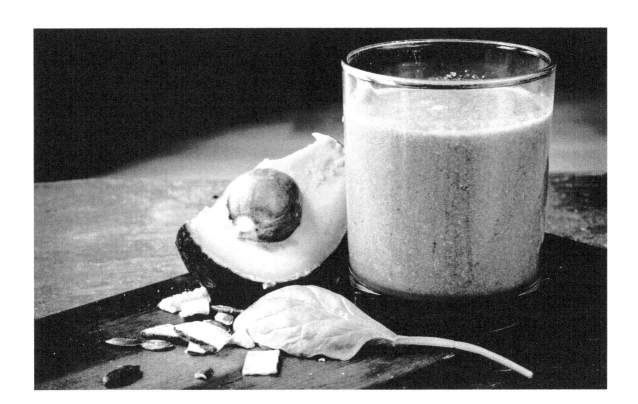

INGREDIENTS

½ cup unsweetened coconut milk
½ tbsp MCT oil or coconut oil
1 scoop collagen protein powder
½ avocado
1 tbsp sunflower seed butter
1 handful of spinach
1 tsp sugar-free vanilla extract
Swerve or sweetener of choice to
taste
½ cup ice cubes

This is how you make the recipe

1. Simply blend together until smooth.
2. Serve and enjoy!

BREAKFAST CHOCOLATE MILKSHAKE

Servings: 1

Nutritional Facts Per Serving:

Net Carbs:	15.25 g	Protein:	6.5 g
Fat:	36 g	Calories:	420 kcal

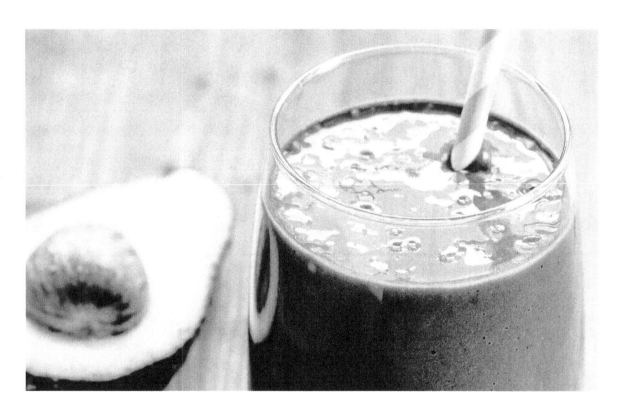

INGREDIENTS

½ cup full-fat coconut milk or heavy cream

½ medium avocado

1-2 tbsp cacao powder

½ tsp sugar-free vanilla extract

Pinch of sea salt

2-4 tbsp Swerve or sweetener of choice

½ cup ice cubes

1 tsp chia seeds

Add water as needed

1 tsp MCT oil

1 scoop collagen peptides (optional)

1 drop mint extract or extract of choice

This is how you make the recipe

1. Add coconut milk, avocado, cacao powder, sugar-free vanilla extract, salt, sweetener and add-ins of choice to a blender. Blend until creamy smooth, using a little water as needed.

2. Add in ice and blend until thick and creamy. Do not over-blend, or you'll lose thickness and coldness.

3. Enjoy right away!

MINT COCO SMOOTHIE

Servings: 2

Nutritional Facts Per Serving:

Net Carbs:	9.07 g	Protein:	17 g
Fat:	49 g	Calories:	561 kcal

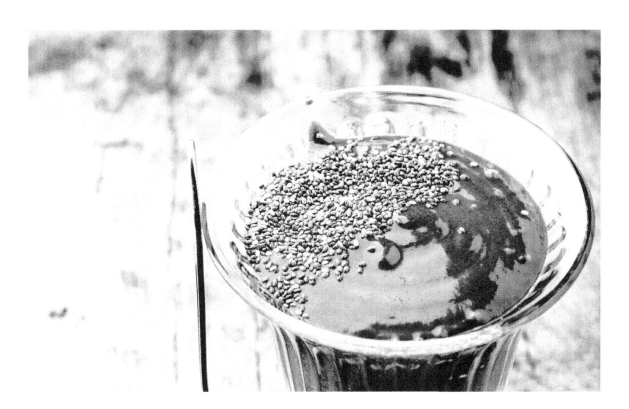

INGREDIENTS

1 cup unsweetened coconut milk

1 cup water

½ cup frozen cauliflower

1 avocado

1 scoop collagen protein

1 tsp sugar-free vanilla extract

1 tbsp chopped mint

1 tbsp cacao powder

1 tbsp coconut oil

Dash of Ceylon cinnamon

Dash of sea salt

Toppings: coconut flakes, chia seeds, flaxseeds, pumpkin seeds, sliced macadamia nuts (optional)

This is how you make the recipe

1. Throw all ingredients into a blender and blend until very smooth and creamy.

2. Serve and enjoy!

NO GUILT CHIA TEA SMOOTHIE

Servings: 1

Nutritional Facts Per Serving:

Net Carbs:	3.2 g	Protein:	15 g
Fat:	12 g	Calories:	179 kcal

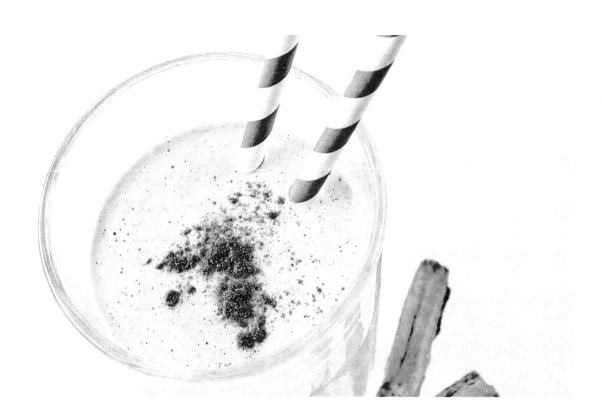

INGREDIENTS

1 cup brewed chia tea

½ cup unsweetened vanilla almond milk

1 scoop unsweetened vanilla protein powder

1 tbsp Swerve or sweetener of choice

1 pinch ground cinnamon

1 cup ice cubes

This is how you make the recipe

1. Combine them all in your blender and blend until smooth!

2. Serve and enjoy!

BLUEBERRY BANANA BREAD SMOOTHIE

Servings: 2

Nutritional Facts Per Serving:

Net Carbs:	4.6 g	Protein:	2.4 g
Fat:	22.5 g	Calories:	235 kcal

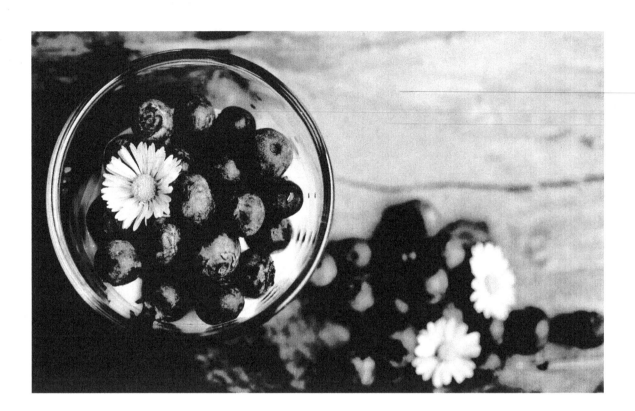

INGREDIENTS

3 tbsp golden flaxseed meal

1 tbsp chia seeds

2 cups vanilla unsweetened coconut milk (from the carton)

2 tbsp Swerve or sweetener of choice

¼ cup blueberries

2 tbsp MCT oil

1 ½ tsp banana extract

¼ tsp xanthan gum

This is how you make the recipe

1. Put 2 cups of unsweetened vanilla coconut milk (from the carton) into a blender with 7 ice cubes, 1 ½ tsp banana extract, and sweetener.

2. Add in ¼ cup blueberries.

3. Measure out 3 tbsp golden flaxseed meal and add it into the mixture.

4. Measure 1 tbsp chia seeds and also add in it. Wait for a few minutes before you blend – then blend for 1-2 minutes or until all ingredients are fully mixed.

5. Measure out into servings and enjoy!

BLACKBERRY CHEESECAKE SMOOTHIE

Servings: 1

Nutritional Facts Per Serving:

Net Carbs:	10.5 g	Protein:	8.5 g
Fat:	51 g	Calories:	546 kcal

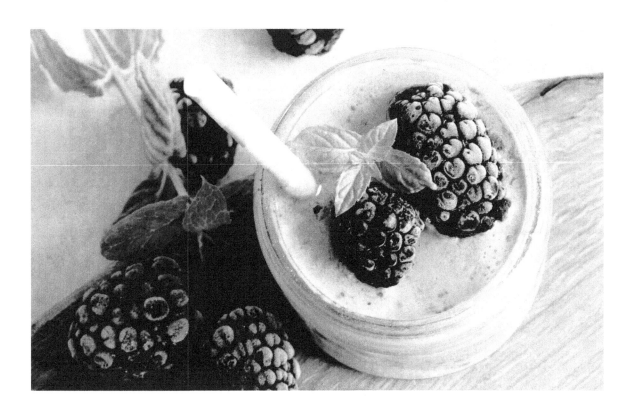

INGREDIENTS

½ cup full-fat cream cheese

1 cup unsweetened almond milk

½ cup blackberries

½ tsp sugar-free vanilla extract

1 tsp Swerve or sweetener of choice

1 tbsp MCT oil (optional)

This is how you make the recipe

1. Add all ingredients to a blender and blend until smooth!

2. Serve and enjoy!

AVOCADO GREEN TEA POWER SHAKE

Servings: 2

Nutritional Facts Per Serving:

Net Carbs:	4 g	Protein:	15 g
Fat:	12.5 g	Calories:	196.5 kcal

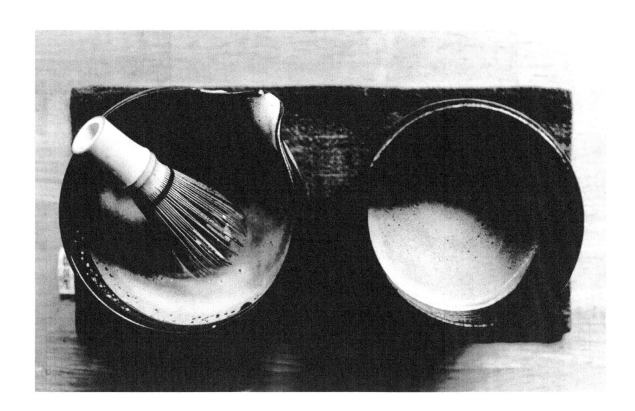

INGREDIENTS

1 tsp matcha green tea powder

1 tbsp hot water

½ medium avocado

½ cup Greek yogurt

¼ cup unsweetened vanilla protein powder

2 tsp Swerve or sweetener of choice

1 ¼ cup unsweetened almond milk

This is how you make the recipe

1. In a small bowl, whisk together matcha powder and hot water. Set aside.

2. Cut avocado into chunks and add to blender. Add yogurt, protein powder, and sweetener.

3. Add almond milk and matcha tea mixture and blend until smooth.

4. Serve and enjoy!

CHOCOLATE PROTEIN SHAKE

Servings: 1

Nutritional Facts Per Serving:

Net Carbs:	14 g	Protein:	11 g
Fat:	24 g	Calories:	357 kcal

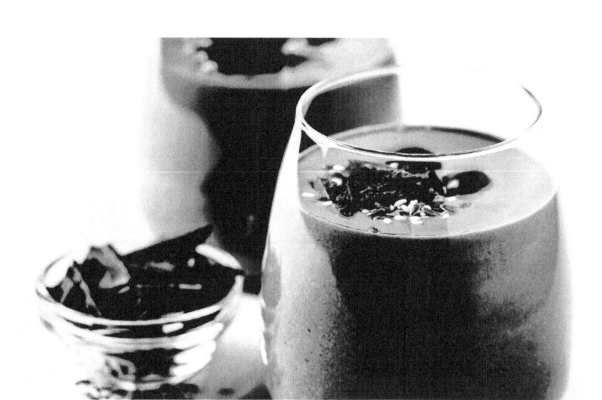

INGREDIENTS

¾ cup almond milk
½ cup ice cubes
2 tbsp unsweetened almond butter
2 tbsp unsweetened cocoa powder
2-3 tbsp Swerve or sweetener of choice
1 tbsp chia seeds, plus more for garnish
½ tbsp sugar-free vanilla extract
Pinch sea salt

This is how you make the recipe

1. Combine all ingredients in blender and blend until smooth.

2. Pour into a glass and garnish with more chia and enjoy!

LEMON COCONUT SMOOTHIE

Servings: 1

Nutritional Facts Per Serving:

Net Carbs:	15.3 g	Protein:	33 g
Fat:	49 g	Calories:	609 kcal

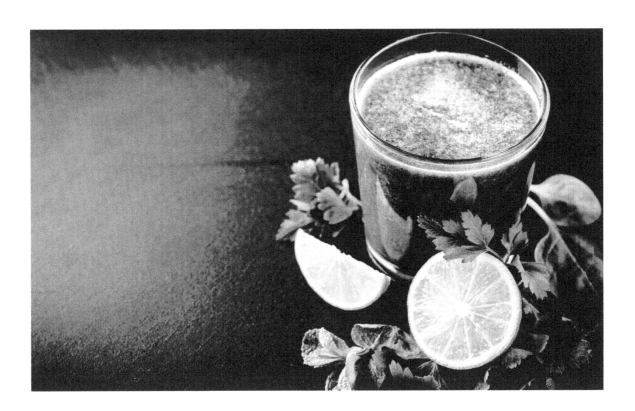

INGREDIENTS

1 lemon, peeled

3 cups baby spinach, washed

2 tbsp raw pumpkin or sunflower seeds

1 cup coconut milk

1 cup water

1 scoop unsweetened protein powder

This is how you make the recipe

1. Blend all the ingredients except the protein until super smooth.

2. Add protein and blend gently until mixed through.

3. Serve and enjoy!

CHOCOLATE RASPBERRY SHAKE

Servings: 1

Nutritional Facts Per Serving:

Net Carbs:	10.3 g	Protein:	6.9 g
Fat:	40 g	Calories:	456 kcal

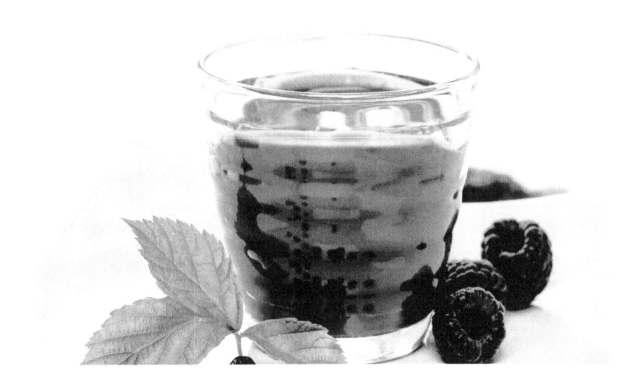

INGREDIENTS

½ cup raspberries

2 scoops unsweetened cocoa powder

1 tbsp chia seeds

1 tbsp heavy cream

1 tbsp coconut oil

1 tbsp cream cheese

1 tsp Swerve or sweetener of choice

¼ cup ice cubes

¾ cup of water

2 tbsp heavy cream (topping)

Pinch of Swerve (garnish)

This is how you make the recipe

1. Add all ingredients to the blender.

2. Blend until thick and smooth.

3. Add a little more water if needed.

4. Topping: Whisk the cream until thick, and pour onto shake with a pinch of Swerve.

5. Enjoy!

KETOGENIC GREEN SMOOTHIE

Servings: 1

Nutritional Facts Per Serving:

Net Carbs:	10.7 g	Protein:	18 g
Fat:	20 g	Calories:	305 kcal

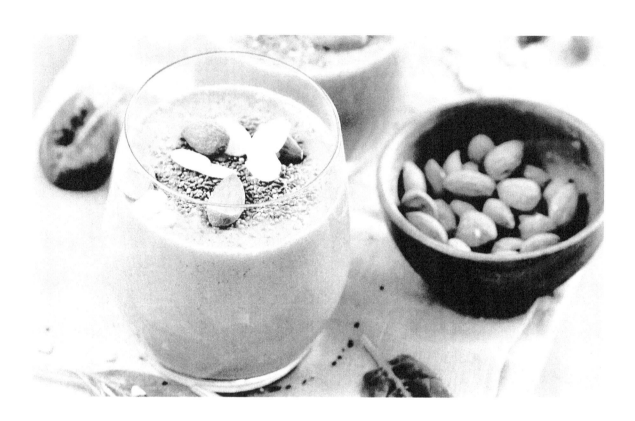

INGREDIENTS

2 cups spinach or kale

10 raw almonds

2 Brazil nuts

1 cup unsweetened coconut milk

1 tbsp psyllium seeds/husks

This is how you make the recipe

1. Place the spinach, almonds, Brazil nuts, and coconut milk into the blender first.

2. Blend until pureed.

3. Add in the rest of the ingredients and blend well.

4. Serve and enjoy!

TURMERIC MILKSHAKE

Servings: 1

Nutritional Facts Per Serving:

Net Carbs:	20 g	Protein:	13 g
Fat:	35 g	Calories:	448 kcal

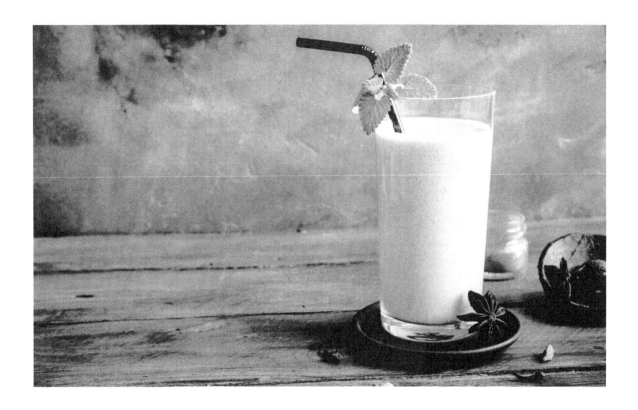

INGREDIENTS

1 ½ cups non-dairy milk

2 tbsp coconut oil

¾ tsp turmeric powder

½ tsp ginger powder

¼ tsp cinnamon

¼ tsp sugar-free vanilla extract

Swerve or sweetener of choice to taste

Pinch sea salt

2 ice cubes

This is how you make the recipe

1. Place all of the ingredients in blender. Blend until thick and golden.

2. Put the turmeric milkshake into a glass and sprinkle with cinnamon and turmeric and enjoy!

PURPLE COW PROTEIN SHAKE

Servings: 1

Nutritional Facts Per Serving:

Net Carbs:	19.4 g	Protein:	4 g
Fat:	4.4 g	Calories:	146 kcal

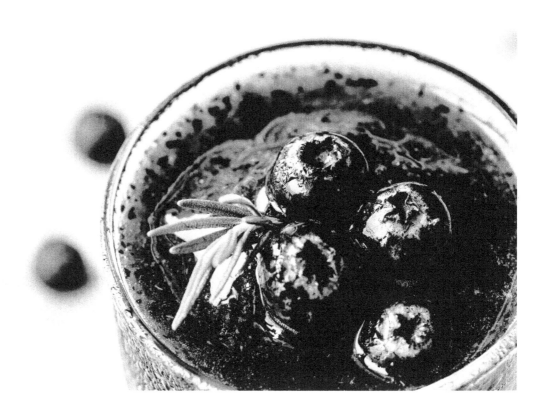

INGREDIENTS

1 cup almond milk

2 tbsp cocoa powder

Handful of fresh strawberries

Handful of fresh blueberries

½ tbsp chia seeds

Nuts, spinach, nut butters, chia seeds (optional)

This is how you make the recipe

1. Simply mix everything in a blender until smooth.

2. Sprinkle with chia seeds.

3. Serve and enjoy!

COCOA COCONUT SHAKE

Servings: 2

Nutritional Facts Per Serving:
Net Carbs:	32.7 g	Protein:	2.75 g
Fat:	28 g	Calories:	391 kcal

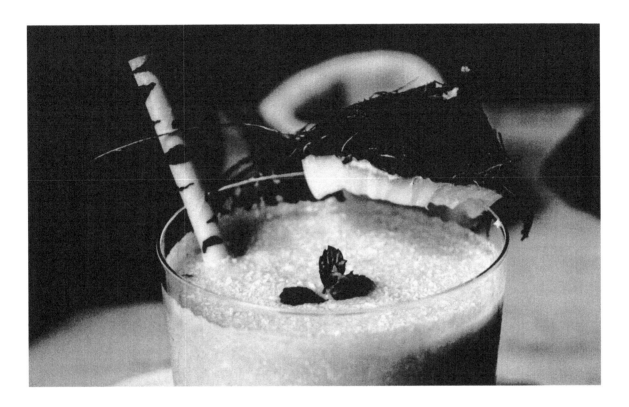

INGREDIENTS

½ cup unsweetened coconut cream

2 tbsp MCT oil or coconut oil (melted)

1 cup almond or unsweetened coconut drinking milk

2 tbsp cocoa powder

Pinch sea salt

½ tbsp creamy almond butter or sunflower seed butter

Swerve, berries, cinnamon to add for sweetness (optional)

This is how you make the recipe

1. Place all ingredients into a blender, blend all together until smooth.

2. Add in sweetener, berries and/or cinnamon to sweeten it up if you wish.

3. Serve and enjoy!

STRAWBERRY MILKSHAKE

Servings: 1

Nutritional Facts Per Serving:

Net Carbs:	12.7 g	Protein:	4.4 g
Fat:	31 g	Calories:	363 kcal

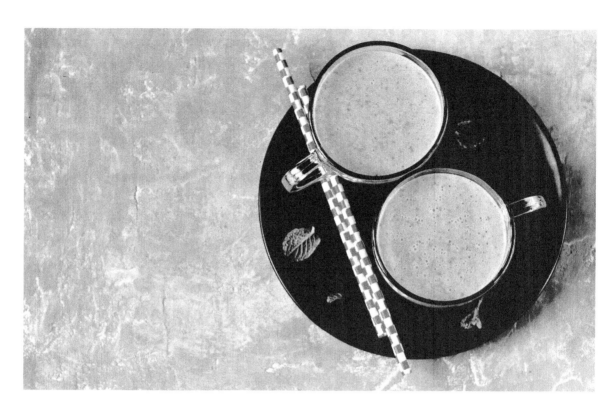

INGREDIENTS

¼ cup coconut milk or heavy whipping cream

¾ cup almond milk or water

½ cup fresh strawberries

1 tbsp MCT oil or coconut oil

½ tsp sugar-free vanilla extract

1 tbsp Swerve or sweetener of choice

1 tbsp chia seeds

Whipped cream or coconut milk (topping)

This is how you make the recipe

1. Place the coconut milk, almond milk, strawberries, MCT oil and sweetener into a blender.

2. Add a tablespoon of chia seeds for a thicker smoothie consistency and pulse until smooth.

3. Serve and enjoy!

AVOCADO BREAKFAST SHAKE

Servings: 1

Nutritional Facts Per Serving:

Net Carbs:	7.4 g	Protein:	10 g
Fat:	25 g	Calories:	319 kcal

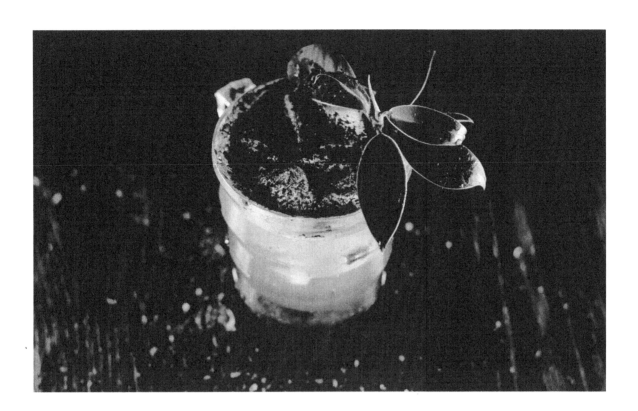

INGREDIENTS

½ avocado

2 cups nut milk

1 tbsp Swerve or sweetener of choice

1 tbsp nut butter

1-2 ice cubes

1 tbsp unsweetened cacao powder

½ tsp sugar-free vanilla extract

1 handful of spinach

This is how you make the recipe

1. Mix all ingredients in a blender and blend until smooth.

2. Serve and enjoy!

CHOCOLATE HAZELNUT SHAKE

Servings: 1

Nutritional Facts Per Serving:

Net Carbs:	21.5 g	Protein:	40 g
Fat:	20 g	Calories:	453 kcal

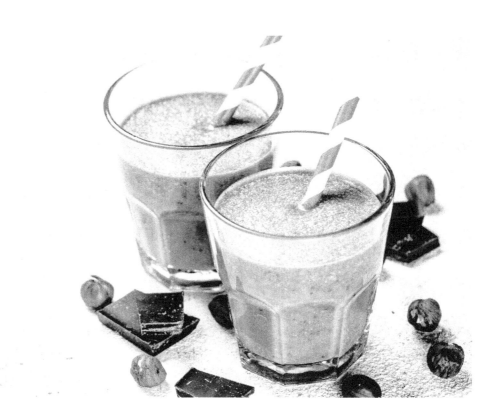

INGREDIENTS

1 cup unsweetened almond milk

1 cup plain double-fermented milk kefir or cottage cheese

½ cup ice cubes

2 tbsp unsweetened cocoa powder

1 ½ tbsp collagen (optional)

1 tbsp Swerve or sweetener of choice

1 tbsp hazelnut extract (to taste)

¼ cup unsweetened protein powder

¼ tsp sea salt

This is how you make the recipe

1. Add all ingredients in blender, blend until smooth.

2. Serve and enjoy!

MATCHA KETOGENIC SMOOTHIE BOWL

Servings: 1

Nutritional Facts Per Serving:

Net Carbs:	17.8 g	Protein:	5.7 g
Fat:	17 g	Calories:	290 kcal

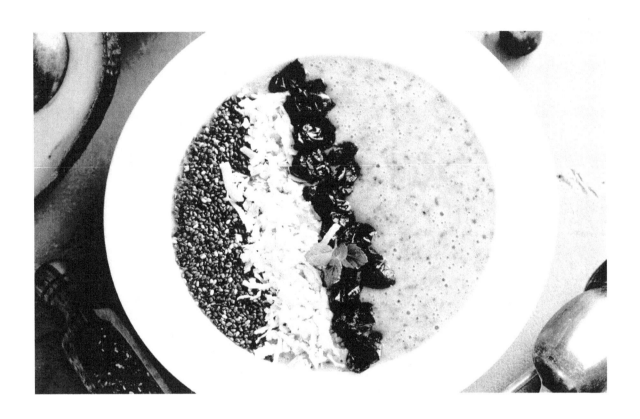

INGREDIENTS

1 tsp matcha powder

1 scoop greens powder (optional)

1 cup coconut yogurt or regular Greek yogurt

1 tbsp chia seeds

1 tbsp goji berries

1 tbsp coconut flakes

1 tbsp cacao nibs

Swerve to taste (optional)

This is how you make the recipe

1. Blend the matcha powder with the yogurt. Add in Swerve to sweeten(optional).

2. Pour the smoothie into a bowl.

3. Top with the chia seeds, goji berries, coconut flakes, and cacao nibs.

4. Enjoy with a spoon.

RASPBERRY PROTEIN SHAKE

Servings: 1

Nutritional Facts Per Serving:

Net Carbs:	8.6 g	Protein:	43 g
Fat:	47 g	Calories:	635 kcal

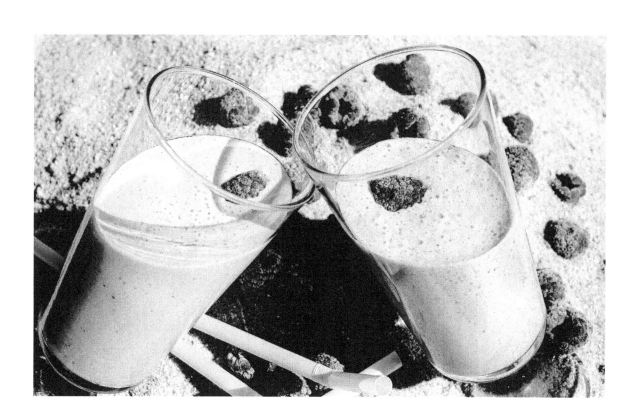

INGREDIENTS

1 cup unsweetened almond milk

½ cup heavy cream

3 tbsp unsweetened protein powder

½ cup fresh raspberries

½ cup ice cubes

1 tsp Swerve or sweetener of choice

This is how you make the recipe

1. Place all ingredients in blender and blend until smooth.

2. Serve and enjoy!

KEY LIME PIE SMOOTHIE

Servings: 2

Nutritional Facts Per Serving:

Net Carbs:	17.3 g	Protein:	19 g
Fat:	75 g	Calories: 802.5 kcal	

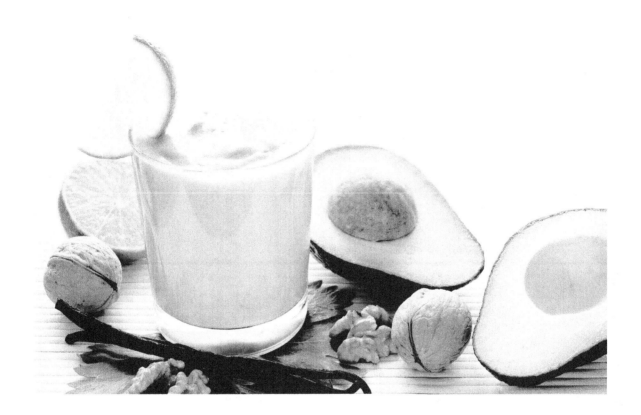

INGREDIENTS

2 cups coconut milk

¼ cup raw cashews, soaked (if you do not have a high power blender to pulverize) or macadamia nuts

4 tbsp lime juice

½ avocado

2 handfuls spinach or any greens

1 tbsp Swerve or sweetener of choice

2 tbsp coconut butter

2 tbsp chia seeds (optional)

2 tbsp collagen

Splash sugar-free vanilla extract (optional)

Zest of one lime to taste (optional)

This is how you make the recipe

1. Place all ingredients into a blender and blend until smooth and creamy.

2. Serve and enjoy!

THICK CHOCOLATE MILKSHAKE

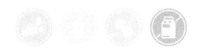

Servings: 1

Nutritional Facts Per Serving:

Net Carbs:	20.2 g	Protein:	6.7 g
Fat:	36 g	Calories:	440 kcal

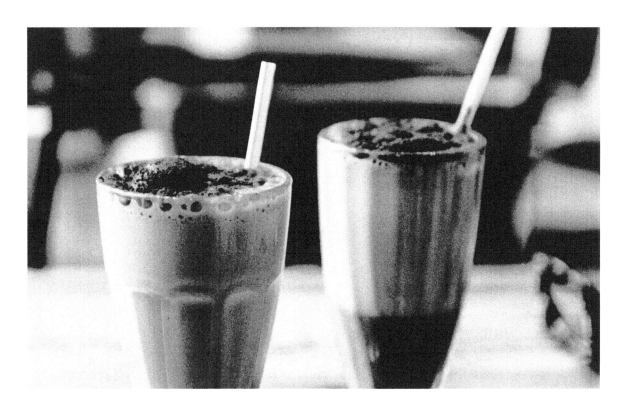

INGREDIENTS

½ cup full-fat coconut milk or heavy cream

½ medium avocado to taste

1-2 tbsp cacao powder to taste

½ tsp sugar-free vanilla extract

Pinch sea salt

2-4 tbsp Swerve or sweetener of choice

½ cup ice cubes

Water as needed

1 tsp chia seeds (optional)

MCT oil or coconut oil (optional)

Collagen peptides (optional)

Mint extract (optional)

This is how you make the recipe

1. Add coconut milk, avocado, cacao powder, sugar-free vanilla extract, salt, sweetener and add-ins of choice to a blender. Blend until creamy smooth, using a little water as needed.

2. Add in ice and blend until it's thick and creamy.

3. Add in chia seeds and plunge until mixed (optional).

4. Serve and enjoy!

Made in the USA
Coppell, TX
10 March 2020

16697759R00050